AIDS-Related Opportunistic Infections

AIDS-Related Opportunistic Infections

Claudia D. Galanda
Editor

Nova Biomedical Books
New York

For permission to use material from this book please contact us:
Telephone 631-231-7269; Fax 631-231-8175
Web Site: http://www.novapublishers.com

Library of Congress Cataloging-in-Publication Data

AIDS-related opportunistic infections / editor, Claudia D. Galanda.
p. ; cm.
Includes bibliographical references and index.
ISBN 978-1-60692-144-9 (hardcover)
1. AIDS (Disease)--Complications. 2. Opportunistic infections. I. Galanda, Claudia D.
[DNLM: 1. AIDS-Related Opportunistic Infections. WC 503.5 A2887 2009]
RA643.8.A36 2009 362.196'9792--dc22
2009000146

Published by Nova Science Publishers, Inc. ✝ New York

Contents

Preface

Chapter I - Background: Induced sputum is a useful technique for assessing airway inflammation, but its role in the diagnosis of lung disease in immunosupressed patients needs further investigation.

Objective: To compare the use of induced sputum and BAL in the diagnosis of infectious lung diseases in HIV positive patients.

Methods: HIV positive patients older than 14 were evaluated at a reference hospital. Patients with respiratory symptoms for seven days or longer, with a normal or abnormal chest x-ray, and those without respiratory symptoms but with an abnormal chest x-ray, were included in the study. All patients were submitted to clinical, radiological and laboratory evaluation, after which induced sputum and bronchoscopy with bronchoalveolar lavage were carried out. The samples were subjected to the following techniques: *Gram* and *Ziehl-Neelsen* staining, quantitative culture growth for pyogenic bacteria, direct staining for fungi, culture growth for mycobacteria and fungi, and *Groccott-Gomori* staining for *Pneumocystis jiroveci*, as well as total and differential cell counts.

Results: The induced sputum sensitivity was 65.9%, specificity 76.9%, predictive positive values 90%, predictive negative value 41.6%, and accuracy 68.5% for the diagnosis of infectious lung diseases in HIV positive patients, compared with BAL.

Conclusion: Based on these data, induced sputum is a useful technique for the diagnosis of infectious lung diseases in HIV patients.

Chapter II - Still in the era of potent, combined antiretroviral therapy, late recognition of HIV disease or lack of sufficient immune recovery pose HIV-infected patients at risk to develop opportunistic infections by atypical mycobacteria, which are environmental organisms commonly retrieved in soil and superficial waters. Among these microorganisms, the most frequent is represented by *Mycobacterium avium-intracellulare* (*Mycobacterium avium-intracellulare* complex, or MAC). Health care professionals who face HIV-infected patients should suspect disseminated mycobacterial disease when a deep immunodeficiency is present, as represented by a CD4+ lymphocyte count below 50-100 cells/μL, and often systemic, non-specific signs and symptoms, and associated non-specific laboratory abnormalities. Mycobacterial culture of peripheral blood is a reliable technique for diagnosing disseminated disease. A set of two cultures may identify over 95% of cases of *Mycobacterium avium-intracellulare* bacteremia. Microscopical examination (Ziehl-Nielsen stain and comparable techniques), and culture biopsies from other normally sterile body sites (i.e. bone marrow, lymph nodes, or liver), also may be useful to pose a diagnosis of AIDS-related mycobacterial disease. Among drugs active against atypical mycobacteria, besides some anti-tubercular compound, the rifampicin derivative rifabutin, and the novel fluoroquinolones, the availability of macrolides greatly contributed to improve both prophylaxis and treatment outcome of disseminated mycobacteriosis complicating the course of AIDS. Although multiple questions remain about which regimens are optimal, general recommendations can be expressed on the ground of existing evidences. Treatment should begin with associated clarithromycin (or azithromycin), plus ethambutol and rifabutin (with the rifabutin dosing depending on other concomitant medications that might result in drug-drug interactions). A combined three-drug regimen is preferred for patients who cannot be prescribed an effective antiretroviral regimen immediately. Patients with a CD4+ lymphocyte count below 50 cells/μL who do not have clinical evidence of active mycobacterial disease, should receive a primary prophylaxis with either clarithromycin or azithromycin; the latter could be coadministered rifabutin. Anti-mycobacterial prophylaxis may be discontinued in patients without a history of recognized mycobacterial disease, whose CD4+ lymphocyte count remains above 100 cells/μL, for at least three months while on combined antiretroviral therapy. With regard to subjects on secondary antimycobacterial prophylaxis, in appears safe to discontinue it when a sustained CD4+ lymphocyte count exceeds at least 100 cells/μL for at least 3-6 consecutive months, during a concurrent, effective antiretroviral regimen.

Chapter III - Pneumocystis pneumonia (PCP) or pneumocystosis remains as one of the most prevalent opportunistic infections in patients infected with the human immunodeficiency virus (HIV) and remains as one of the most common causes death in patients with AIDS. Pneumocystosis in humans is caused by to *P. jiroveci*, different from *P. carinii* that is one of the two *Pneumocystis* species found only in rats. First was identified as a protozoan nearly 100 years ago, it has been reclassified as a fungus, in 1988, based on DNA analysis. *P. jiroveci* has worldwide distribution among humans and has been detected in a variety of animals. It is difficult to find in the environment and has not been found in nonhuman hosts. It is absent or present a very low levels in healthy adults, in contrast, it is fairly common in immunocompromised individuals. *Pneumocystis* is acquired by airborne route and takes up residence in the alveoli adhering to type I cells. In immunocompromised hosts it propagates and fills the alveoli. It results in increased alveolar-capillary permeability and damage to type I cells. There is alteration on the pulmonary surfactant and, in severe disease, may include interstitial edema, fibrosis, and hyaline membrane formation. The clinical picture is quite variable. Most patients are usually ill for two to three weeks. Progressive dyspnea is characteristic, but dry cough, tachycardia, tachypnea, cyanosis, and low-grade fever are also common manifestations. Lung auscultation is usually unremarkable. Arterial blood gas demonstrates hypoxia, increased alveolar-arterial gradient and respiratory alkalosis. Desaturation on exercise of $\geq$ 5% is a reliable and quick test. Chest radiography classically shows fine, bilateral, diffuse infiltrates beginning in the perihilar regions. Early in the disease the chest radiography may be normal. Other presentations include unilateral infiltrates, cavitary lesions, nodular densities, cystic formation, pleural effusion, pneumothorax, and pneumomediastinum. High resolution computerized tomography is more sensitive than chest radiography in the diagnosis of PCP. Definitive diagnosis is based on specific identification of the organism by histopathologic staining. Sputum induction has wide variety of success. In seven prospective studies demonstrated 55.5% sensitivity and 98.6% specificity. Fiber optic bronchoscopy with bronchoalveolar lavage has > 90% sensitivity and 100% specificity. The drug of choice is trimethoprim-sulfamethoxazole (TMP-SMZ) and in severe cases it is recommended the concomitant use of steroids. Alternative drugs include: Atovaquone, clindamycin, primaquine, dapsone plus trimethoprim and pentamidine

Chapter IV - In recent years, we have observed that *Pneumocystis* pneumonia (PcP) is frequently super-infected by trichomonads, whereas PcP was thought to be a single opportunistic infection caused by *Pneumocystis jirovecii.* Moreover, in cases rich in *Pneumocystis* organisms, the frequency of coinfection with trichomonads in alveoli can reach 100%. On the other hand, we have observed that super-infection by trichomonads could develop as well in immunocompetent patients, for instance in the course of acute respiratory distress syndrome (ARDS). This latter finding reinforces the view that in PcP trichomonads express a peculiar form of opportunism, where local conditions in alveolar lumens play a major role instead of immunodeficiency. Trichomonads development could be a secondary event in alveoli filled by *Pneumocystis*, and eradication of the fungus should therefore be followed by elimination of protists. Thus, these data could not have implications in patient management. However, they raise many questions in several fields that are examined in this Commentary: a) questions about the delay of such a report since the start of the AIDS epidemic, b) questions about the source of trichomonads and species involved, and c) questions about the role of trichomonads in PcP and their potential deleterious effect. Data about trichomonads found in the course of PcP are mainly observational. Nevertheless, currently proposed pathophysiological conceptions of PcP could be reconsidered in the future at the levels of both clinical and biological research.

Chapter V - HIV-infected children are susceptible to opportunistic infections (OIs) due to immune suppression stage caused by HIV. Before the availability of antiretroviral therapy (ART), the common OIs among children were serious bacterial infections, *Pneumocystis jiroveci* pneumonia (PCP), candidiasis, herpes zoster, tuberculosis, disseminated *Mycobacterium avium* complex (MAC), and systemic fungal infection. Antiretroviral drugs control HIV viral replication and restore immune function. In the era of antiretroviral therapy, there is a significant reduction in rate of OIs which leads to reduction of morbidity and mortality in HIV-infected children. After HIV-infected children gain CD4 cell recovery while receiving stable antiretroviral therapy, opportunistic infection prophylaxis such as cotrimoxazole for PCP prophylaxis can be discontinued safely. In this article the perspectives of opportunistic infections management including immune reconstitution inflammatory syndrome and when to discontinue prophylaxis in the era of active antiretroviral therapy will be described.

Chapter VI - Opportunistic infection is a problem in managing immunodeficiency virus (HIV) infection with severely impaired immune status. A number of infections are documented and more knowledge is required for proper management. At present, HIV infection has a very high prevalence in many tropical developing countries. An important concern is tropical blood infection, which is also common in these countries. A high chance of co-occurrence can be seen. A compelling question remains regarding whether there is any specific implication for the finding of co-occurrence of HIV and tropical blood infections. There is some new recent evidence for opportunistic infection in those co-occurrence cases. In this chapter, the author summarizes tropical blood infection in HIV and further extrapolates to discuss the role of blood infection as opportunistic infection or a strong supporting factor for the vulnerability of HIV-infected patients to opportunistic infection.

Chapter VII - Opportunistic infection is an important complication in the course of human immunodeficiency virus (HIV) infection. Opportunistic infection is common for the HIV-infected cases with impaired immune status. A number of infections have been documented and are the focus in HIV medicine. Although the pattern of opportunistic infections in different parts of the world share some common characteristics, the difference among various regions is still an area of interest at present. In this work, the author summarized reports from Thailand on oppportunistic infection in HIV infection. The four main groups of opportunistic infections are the focus of this chapter: respiratory tract infections, neurological infections, skin infections and gastrointestinal infections. It can be shown that opportunistic infection is important in coping with HIV-infected cases in Thailand. In addition, practitioners who deal with patients from Thailand and nearby tropical countries should be aware of the significance of tropical infections as opportunistic infections in HIV-infected cases in Thailand.

Chapter VIII - The immune surveillance hypothesis of cancer emerged during the twentieth century but until recently there have been few clinical examples of immunoprevention of malignancy. The worldwide epidemic of the human immunodeficiency virus (HIV) represent the most striking example of genome emergence, transmission and expansion. Concomitantly, the field of anti-retroviral therapy has witnessed remarkable progress and there are now over fifteen approved therapeutic agents for treatment of this pathogen that once caused a uniformly fatal illness. With longer term follow-up, we also observe that the anti-retroviral induced maintenance of immunocompetence, also prevents common HIV-related malignancies. This is discussed below with specific reference to effective anti-retroviral therapy preventing both Kaposi's sarcoma and non Hodgkin's lymphoma in advanced HIV disease.

Chapter IX - in common a similar histopathology and expression of human herpes virus 8 (HHV-8) in the lesions. Two forms are associated with immune suppression, post-transplant KS and AIDS-related KS, while the two others, classic KS and African endemic KS are not. HHV-8 infections are normally benign, with the incidence of HHV-8 infection being much higher than the incidence of KS. The cellular deregulation that leads to the formation of KS lesions is poorly understood, as is the infected cell type. It is also unknown whether gene expression patterns are similar between the epidemiological forms, especially as two forms are not associated with immune dysfunction. To gain insight into the genes expressed in KS lesions, we have generated Serial Analysis of Gene Expression (SAGE) libraries from both AIDS-KS and African endemic KS tissue to analyze mRNA levels in KS. The SAGE libraries were compared with each other and with libraries in the SAGEmap database. Systematic analysis of the level of gene expression of twelve specific gene families or related genes, including HHV-8 genes, was performed for both endemic KS and AIDS-KS tissue. The results suggested that endemic KS and AIDS-KS have a similar pattern of gene expression, in line with their comparable histopathology.

High or very high expression was found in KS compared with other libraries for psoriasin, HLA-C, complement component 1, keratin 16, galectin 9, plexin D1, CD51, CD31, CCL18, CCL19, CCL21, and many other genes. In general, not the tag counts but rather the tag count ratio of KS versus other libraries gave information about the level of gene expression. Interestingly, a few genes were overexpressed in AIDS-KS compared with endemic KS (e.g. Von Willebrand Factor, D component of complement), while others were overexpressed in endemic KS (e.g. HLA-F, MMP-12, CD74, calgranulin-A). It has been suggested that iron is an important factor in the establishment of KS. Analysis of iron-related gene expression in KS, however, suggested no clear abnormalities. Relatively high expression was only found for the light polypeptide of ferritin, and heme oxygenase-1, and intermediate expression was seen for the hemoglobin scavenger receptor CD163, compatible with macrophage-related iron-uptake as erythrocytes leak from abnormal vessels in the KS lesions.

In conclusion, the comparison of gene family expression in KS SAGE libraries has provided new insights into the molecular mechanism involved in the pathogenesis of KS.

Chapter X - In Africa, it was very common that older family members make important health decisions when young members are sick (Seeley, Kajura, Bachengama, Okongo, Wagner, & Mulder, 1993; Foster 2000). Traditionally, the extended family and clan had been the backbone of the African family system as they had provided help and support to its members whenever needed, especially in times of crises (Foster, 2000). However, because of the unprecedented demands and needs of people living with HIV/AIDS, these institutions may not be able to meet these challenges.

Additionally, because of modernization and individualism prevalent in urban areas, the roles of the extended family in times of need may be weakened (Foster & Williamson, 2000). In fact, AIDS is an exorbitant disease, and currently, most Africans cannot afford effective antiviral therapies. Some families have spent their life savings on loved ones with AIDS but have not seen any improvement in the health of the sick (Moore & Henry, 2005; Family Health International, 2001; UNICEF, 2002). Also, stigma associated with HIV/AIDS has made it difficult for family members to cope with the disease and openly talk about their loved ones who are either HIV positive or have AIDS. Consequently, extended family members or clans may be reluctant to help because of fear of being stigmatized or the inability to care for a sick family or provide assistance because of poverty.

In: AIDS-Related Opportunistic Infections
Editor: Claudia D. Galanda
ISBN: 978-1-60692-144-9

Chapter I

Induced Sputum versus Bronchoalveolar Lavage in the Diagnosis of Infectious Lung Diseases in Human Immunodeficiency Virus-Positive Patients

Rosemeri Maurici da Silva[1]
[1]University of Southern Santa Catarina (UNISUL), Florianopolis, Santa Catarina, Brazil

Abstract

Background: Induced sputum is a useful technique for assessing airway inflammation, but its role in the diagnosis of lung disease in immunosupressed patients needs further investigation.
Objective: To compare the use of induced sputum and BAL in the diagnosis of infectious lung diseases in HIV positive patients.
Methods: HIV positive patients older than 14 were evaluated at a reference hospital. Patients with respiratory symptoms for seven days or longer, with a normal or abnormal chest x-ray, and those without respiratory symptoms but with an abnormal chest x-ray, were included in the study. All patients were submitted to clinical, radiological and laboratory evaluation, after which induced sputum and bronchoscopy with bronchoalveolar lavage were carried out. The samples were subjected to the following techniques: *Gram* and *Ziehl-Neelsen* staining, quantitative culture growth for pyogenic bacteria, direct staining for fungi, culture growth for mycobacteria and fungi, and *Groccott-Gomori* staining for *Pneumocystis jiroveci*, as well as total and differential cell counts.
Results: The induced sputum sensitivity was 65.9%, specificity 76.9%, predictive positive values 90%, predictive negative value 41.6%, and accuracy 68.5% for the diagnosis of infectious lung diseases in HIV positive patients, compared with BAL.

Conclusion: Based on these data, induced sputum is a useful technique for the diagnosis of infectious lung diseases in HIV patients.

Introduction

According to the latest estimates, 33.2 million individuals now live with AIDS worldwide and 2.1 million suffered from the disease in 2007. The situation is not different from the global epidemic in Latin American countries, where 1.6 million individuals are now living with AIDS. [1]

With the introduction of combined retroviral therapy, attention to preventive work and treatment of clinical intercurrences, there is a growing increase in survival and a statistically significant drop of almost all opportunistic diseases. [2]

The main characteristic of the retrovirus that causes AIDs, known as human immunodeficiency virus (HIV), is infection of $CD4^{+}$ (LT4) lymphocytes or helper cells, and macrophages. Such infection results in a progressive decrease in the number and function of LT4, with consequent impairment of cellular immunity. This disturbance in cellular immunity causes the person to become susceptible to a series of opportunistic infections and neoplastic processes. These immunity alterations vary according to the disease stage or the duration of host infection. Even though cellular immunity is primarily affected, other defects are also perceived and play an important role in morbimortality. T lymphocytes are critical for the activation of B lymphocytes and the subsequent production of immunoglobulines, which is jeopardized by the primary disorder of cellular immunity. In addition, functional defects in B lymphocytes are observed, with progressive loss of specific immunoglobulin response. These systemic alterations are concomitant with local alterations. For example, the respiratory tract, which has alveolar macrophages, lymphocytes, and polymorphonuclear lymphocytes as important lines of defense, is widely susceptible to a series of clinical conditions. The macrophages present CD4 antigens can be directly infected by HIV. Besides compromising the cell defense response, the infection in not cytopathic immediately, functioning as viral reservoir. The chimiotaxis is also disturbed, which results in a decrease or even absence of granulamatosis. In parallel, there is also a chimiotaxis decrease for polymorphonuclear lymphocytes. These disarrangements predispose individuals to opportunistic infections not only dependent on impaired cellular defense, but also facilitate infection from organisms that depend primarily on humoral defenses. This concept becomes important due to the fact that the etiologic spectrum of diseases, when analyzed under such an approach, becomes practically infinite. [3]

Infectious and neoplastic complications are the most important causes of morbimortality in HIV infected patients. A great number of them are shown as pulmonary disease, which entail a major impact on the survival and quality of life of these patients. It is estimated that in 65% of infected patients with HIV, the pulmonary system is the site of the first clinical manifestation of the syndrome, and that 80% of these individuals have pulmonary manifestation in the course of their lung disease. [4] Assessing 1,067 patients with AIDS, Murray and colleagues found that 41% of these had lung problems. [5] In a period of four years observing 130 patients with AIDS, Stover and collaborators described that 47% of these patients had pulmonary disorders. [6] With the introduction of combined antiretroviral therapy, there was a gradual decrease in morbidity and mortality of the disease, resulting from the viral load decrease and the increase in $CD4^+$ cell count. This effect is due to the decrease in the occurrence of various opportunistic infections, including tuberculosis and pneumocistosis. [7,8] This observation is supported by the fact that the number of bronchoscopies and pulmonary infections that require bronchoscopy have been declining since 1990, which coincides with the period of the introduction of the new therapeutic modality. [9]

The respiratory infection manifestations in patients with AIDS may be caused by any group of pathogens, besides the fact that infection with HIV is a dynamic condition in which the immune status and the risk for specific etiological agents change with the time and the stage of the disease. [10]

Pneumocistosis, whose causative agent is *Pneumocystis jiroveci*, is one of the most prevalent conditions. Until 1980, the agent causing pneumocistosis was considered a protozoan, and only since 1988 has been classified as a fungus. Recently, it was observed that the organisms of the *Pneumocystis* genus that cause disease in various species have different DNA sequences; thus, a change in nomenclature for the organisms that infect the human species for *Pneumocystis jiroveci* was proposed, leaving the term *carinii* reserved for other species. [11]

Pneumocistosis is characterized by the insidious or sudden start of dyspnea and dry cough, accompanied by perihilar reticular or reticulonodular infiltrates in chest radiograms, which may progress in a few days to diffuse air-space consolidation. The physical examination in most cases is normal, and, in 10% of cases, there is no radiologic change. [12]

Other fungi also infect this group of patients, and the lung disease typically accompanies the disease spread. The relapses are frequent despite treatment and prophylaxis becomes imperative. Another important feature is the high density of microorganisms in injuries and poor formation of granuloms. [12,13,14] Radiologically they appear as pleural effusion, mediastinal adenomegaly, diffuse infiltrates or nodules, and absence of image change can also be observed. In the cryptococcosis, whose causative agent is the *Criptococcus neoformans* (*gatti* or *grubii* variety), meningitis is the most common manifestation, although the lung is also affected with some frequency. [13,14] Histoplasmosis, caused by *Histoplasma capsulatum*, most commonly affects the lungs. The radiographic examination may be normal in up to 35% of cases. Other less common agents include *Coccidioides immitis*, *Candida sp.* and *Paracoccidioides brasiliensis*. [8,13,14]

Cytomegalovirus causes retinitis in 5% of cases, and with less frequency may be responsible for pneumonitis. This agent has been isolated in the bronchoalveolar lavage or sputum in 30 to 40% of patients with pneumonia caused by other etiologies, and its role as a cause of lung disease is linked to the need for its isolation in tissue samples. [8,13,14]

Currently, bacterial pneumonia has overcome pneumocistosis in terms of frequency in some reports. The presence of more than two episodes of bacterial pneumonia in one year is a diagnostic criterion for AIDS. [15] The most common agents are *Streptococcus pneumoniae*, *Haemophilus influenzae* and *Staphylococcus aureus*, although any bacteria can be described in this group of patients. [16] Bacterial pneumonia, acquired in the community and caused by

Streptococcus pneumonia, shows rates around 18 cases per 1,000 patients per year, five times the rate found in immunocompetent patients. [13,14]

Pulmonary tuberculosis plays an important role in pulmonary infections in this group, especially in countries where the prevalence of this disease is high. Around 8% of patients diagnosed with active tuberculosis are co-infected with HIV. [8] The disease radiological and clinical pattern reflects the extent of the immune compromised system, and the typical forms with cavitation and affection of superior lobules are infrequent. The most common is mediastinal adenopathy and diffuse non-cavity infiltrates. [12] Other mycobacteria such as *Mycobacterium avium* complex, account for a smaller number of cases. [8]

Toxoplasmosis, which etiologic agent is *Toxoplasma gondii,* invariably appears as a disease of the central nervous system, but the respiratory tract can also be affected. Lung diseases by *Strongyloides stercoralis* are described as well. [13,14]

Non-infectious diseases respond by the remaining cases of pulmonary affection and include the Kaposi's sarcoma, lymphoma, lung primary neoplasia, lymphoid interstitial pneumonitis and nonspecific interstitial pneumonitis. [17]

The clinical spectrum of lung diseases is very similar to the different etiological agents, making it very difficult to diagnose based on signs and symptoms only. [13,14,18] Although some conditions are found with greater frequency related to immune impairment, which can be monitored by $CD4^+$ cell count, different pathogens can be found in varied cell count. This fact requires great care in interpreting these figures as the sole parameter for risk of lung disease. [19] Similarly, careful interpretation of radiological exams should be carried out, since it also varies for each etiological agent, depending on the degree of immunosuppression. Even correlating radiological aspects with $CD4^+$ cell count, the number of diagnostic possibilities for each category of patients is still multiple. [20] It is known that AIDS infected patients may have radiological changes without concomitant clinical manifestation, and that the incidence of infectious diseases in this group of patients, particularly pulmonary tuberculosis and infection by nontuberculous mycobacteria, is high. [21] There is also the possibility of multiple infections in a single patient, with the presence of two or even more pathogens. [22]

The need for this group of patients to have specific treatment is justified by its high rate of morbidity and mortality. In a study of necropsies, 85% of cases demonstrated one or more respiratory disease as a direct cause of death. [23] Immunoimpaired patients are those with clinical potential for rapid deterioration; the response to treatment is usually delayed in relation to immunocompetent and the toxic reactions to the use of medications are more common and severe. [24,25] It is known that the early establishment of specific and appropriate therapy increases the possibility of success and reduces toxicity. [25] In addition, the empirical treatment can result in loss of the diagnostic opportunity and, consequently, the possibility of effective treatment, influencing the morbimortality and quality of life of these patients, which turns the correct etiologic diagnosis an irreplaceable element in terms of prognosis. Additionally, it is known that the presence of multiple microorganisms decreases the survival, and that the correct treatment of concurrent infections has important prognosis role in the short and long term. [26]

The diagnosis based on signs, symptoms and radiological aspects, as reported earlier, does not allow the presumption of the causative agent, becoming a hard and fruitless exercise. Thus, the respiratory secretions are the ideal material to be examined to search for the infectious agent, and, for that purpose, there are invasive and noninvasive collection techniques.

Among the invasive collection techniques, there are the bronchoscopy with bronchoalveolar lavage and transbronchial pulmonary biopsy, open lung biopsy, the transcutaneous aspiration pulmonary puncture, mediastinoscopy, and pleural puncture biopsy. [10]

Among the non-invasive techniques, there are the serologies, cutaneous tests, blood cultures, and analysis of sputum.

There is still much controversy over the handling of immunocompromised patients and lung diseases, perhaps by the fact that there is not a diagnostic study that alone can identify the causative agent in a consistent manner. Despite all efforts, approximately 50% of patients remain without diagnosis. [27,28]

Hemocultures have low sensitivity but high specificity, which justifies its routine use mainly in immunocompromised patients. [27]

Thoracentesis with pleural biopsy should be performed whenever there is significant pleural effusion. The efficiency of this diagnostic modality in the identification of pathogens is low, but shows high specificity. [27]

Bronchoscopy with bronchoalveolar lavage and transbronchial lung biopsy is considered the next step to the analysis of sputum. The sensitivity of the bronchoalveolar lavage for infectious agents is 38% to 58%, and specificity is 85% or higher. For the diagnosis of bacterial pneumonia, the cut-off point of 10^4 cfu/ml in bronchoalveolar lavage is considered significant and capable of differentiating colonization of infection. [27] The use of routine transbronchial lung biopsy offers few additional data and should be reserved for patients whose bronchoalveolar lavage was not effective in revealing the etiology of the process, besides providing a sample of few cells in comparison with the bronchoalveolar lavage covering more than one million of them. [24,28] Furthermore, transbronchial lung biopsy increases the rate of complications and the procedure is contraindicated in patients with coagulopathies and severe hypoxemia. [24,29]

The transcutaneous transthoracic needle aspiration, described for the first time in 1883, is used in the investigation of focal lesions or peripheral masses where the other diagnostic modalities were unsuccessful. [28] For common bacteria it shows from 33% to 88% of sensitivity and 75% of specificity. [27] Most important complications include pneumothorax, which occurs in approximately 10% of cases, hemoptysis in 1% to 5% of cases, and gas embolism. [30]

Open lung biopsy is indicated in cases of diffuse injuries and presents excellent quality material for histopathology and microbiological tests. Its disadvantage is the high degree of invasiveness and the potential for complications, apart from not being cost-effective to be performed routinely. [27]

The analysis of sputum is the least invasive method available and can have its diagnostic accuracy increased when interpreted in accordance with specific criteria. It is known that the lower respiratory tract is virtually barren, but when the individual expectorates, this material enters in contact with oropharyngeal secretions, nasal and oral, becoming potentially contaminated with microorganisms of the resident microbiota. [31] This problem can be minimized if the collection of material is supervised and if representative criteria of lower airways and absence of significant contamination with the material of the upper respiratory tract are adopted. This goal is achieved when the sample contains less than 10 squamous epithelial cells, more than 25 neutrophils per highly augmented field, and presence of alveolar macrophages. It is known that approximately 25% of sputum samples sent to laboratories for culture are inadequate, leading to great variability and low reliability in the results. [30]

Gram staining method, described in 1883, is useful when it shows a predominant bacterial morphotype and is interpreted in parallel with the culture. The great problem of cultures of sputum is the differentiation between colonization and contamination of the infection itself. The use of quantitative cultures is a viable alternative for this differentiation, since they show high specificity and make the colonization less likely when above a certain cutpoint. An etiological role can be assigned to the microorganism identified in high concentrations and a contaminant role when present in low concentrations. [16,32,33,34] The quantitative cultures differentiate colonizer infecting organisms when more than 10^6 cfu/ml. [30] A positive clinical correlation with the concentration of bacteria can also be observed, and the samples with higher rates present in patients with clinical manifestations are more evident. [34]

Serology and skin tests have limited value in immunocompromised patients. [30]

New laboratory techniques such as polymerase chain reaction and others significantly augment the diagnostic sensitivity, but require highly skilled technical personnel and have additional cost. [18]

The signs and symptoms more frequently found in this group of patients are fever and unproductive cough. The fact that most patients who do not produce sputum spontaneously hampers the initial non-invasive approach, which would be the analysis of sputum. [24] For those individuals who do not have spontaneous expectoration, a method of collection called induced sputum can be used. This technique was initially described in 1958 by Bickerman, Sproul and Barach who introduced a method to induce the production of sputum by inhalation of heated hypertonic aerosol. In 1968, publications already highlighted the concept that this new method was of unique value for the diagnosis of lung diseases in people who did not produce spontaneous expectoration, especially in diseases such as tuberculosis and bacterial pneumonia. [35] The induction of sputum is based on the concept that changes in the microenvironment of the airways, such as the pH and osmolarity, as well as the activation of inflammatory mediators, can sharply increase the secretion and make it possible to obtain samples of this material in patients who originally revealed unproductive cough. [36] It is also a technical collection of simple, low cost and with low rate of complications, most of them being temporary and not serious. [37]

Nowadays, it has been widely used in the monitoring of inflammation of airways, especially in individuals with bronchial asthma. It is a technique that shows promising results in the assessment of diffuse interstitial diseases such as idiopathic pulmonary fibrosis, pneumonites by hypersensitivity and sarcoidosis, but its diagnostic role still needs to be better defined. [38] Similarly, its importance as a diagnostic tool in immunocompromised patients still needs further definition. [28] For some pathogens such as *Pneumocystis jiroveci*, and *Mycobacterium tuberculosis*, this method of collection has proved useful, sensitive and specific, however, for other pathogens its usefulness remains unclear. [39,40,41,42] Pitchenik and collaborators showed a positive reaction to *Pneumocystis jiroveci* around 55%. [40] For the same pathogen, Bigby and collaborators found a sensitivity of 56% and a negative predictive value of 39%. [41] Other studies have shown a sensitivity of 74% and a negative predictive value of 58%. [43] For the same etiological agent, some researchers have not found such satisfactory results. In a study by Rolston and collaborators, only 28% of pneumocistosis cases could be diagnosed by examining the induced sputum. [44] A low yield for the diagnosis of pneumocistosis and other pathogens was also described by Miller and colleagues. [45] For the isolation of *Mycobacterium tuberculosis* a sensitivity of 87% and negative predictive value of 96% was reported. [46] Conde and colleagues described sensitivity of 60%, using culture for *Mycobacterium tuberculosis*. [42] Weinberg and collaborators reached a 40% yield for *Pneumocystis jiroveci* and 10% for *Mycobacterium tuberculosis*. [47]

It is known that invasive procedures are not entirely free of risk, and that patients with AIDS have a better chance than immunocompetent individuals to develop adverse effects through the diagnostic or therapeutic procedures because of their physical weakness and abnormal immune status. [48] An ideal test should have high sensitivity and specificity, high predictive positive and negative value, rapid return, be reproducible, have easy implementation and low cost as primary features. [27] These factors lead to the need to define the exact role of non-invasive techniques, which can be carried out as fast, secure, accessible in institutions in which examinations of high complexity are not widely available, low cost, and with acceptable diagnostic yield. Among the non-invasive procedures, the induction of sputum has shown to be a promising method to comply with the requirements listed above.

As the result of treating these patients and their survival depends on the correct diagnosis of the etiologic agents as well as the optimization of procedures with respect to its invasiveness, cost and speed, we decided to carry out a study in a reference hospital for treatment of patients with HIV/AIDS on the accuracy of the induced sputum examination in the etiological diagnosis of lung infections, comparing its yield with that obtained by bronchoalveolar lavage.

Objective

To compare the yield of induced sputum examination with bronchoalveolar lavage in diagnosing lung infections in human immunodeficiency virus positive patients.

Methods

From the 1st January 2001 to 30th December 2002, all patients aged over 14 years, infected with human immunodeficiency virus (HIV), admitted in a reference hospital for treatment of HIV-positive patients in southern Brazil were evaluated. Individuals with clinical symptoms of the respiratory tract for at least seven days, associated or not with radiological signs of lung disease were included in the study. Also included were those individuals with asymptomatic respiratory problems who showed radiologic lung alterations. [21]

The exclusion criteria were: a) empirical treatment for pulmonary condition for more than a week, [49] b) use of prophylactic treatment for tuberculosis in the last six months and/or *Pneumocystis jiroveci* pneumonia for the past 30 days in relation to the date of admission, [15] c) cachexia and general condition impairment reflected by a Karnofsky index between 20 and 30; [50,51] d) consciousness alteration (obnubilation or coma), [29] and) oxygen partial pressure <80 mmHg, receiving supplementary oxygen through nasal catheter, with 2 liter flow per minute, [29] f) fall in FEV1 greater than 20% during the induction of sputum and/or signs and symptoms that counterindicated the procedure, [52] g) non effective sputum induction; h) refusal to participate in the study, or non-cooperation with the diagnostic procedures.

All patients who complied with the inclusion criteria were invited to participate, received orientation regarding the study and diagnostic techniques, and signed a term of free and informed consent. After this procedure, all patients were submitted to clinical, radiological and laboratory evaluation, being registered in inclusion files, after which sputum induction and bronchoscopy with bronchoalveolar lavage were carried out, with an interval of 24 hours between the two procedures.

The research project was submitted to and approved by the Ethics Committee of the reference hospital.

Clinical, Laboratory and Radiological Methods

Clinical observation consisted of recording the presence of respiratory signs and/or symptoms through structured questionnaire, and the estimated Karnofsky rate. [50] All patients included in the study performed posterior-up and lateral chest X-rays, and computed tomography of chest and mediastinum. Later, participants performed laboratory tests, which included arterial gasometry and lymphocyte CD4+ T-cells count. Arterial blood gasometry was initially held in open air. When the partial pressure of oxygen was at or below 60 mmHg, gasometry was repeated with the patient receiving oxygen through nasal catheter, at 2 liter flow per minute.

Sputum Induction Technique

The induction of sputum was performed using a US-800 Air Standard® nebulizer with nebulization rate of 1 ml/minute ± 0.2 and size of particles specified by the manufacturer between 0.5 to 10 micrometers; and a Microlab 3500® spirometer, obeying the following protocol: [52]

1) Store saline solution in the refrigerator for 15 minutes before use.
2) Inform the patient of the purpose of the procedure and how it will be carried out.
3) Measure basal FEV1 and FVC.

4) Administer 200 μg of inhaled beta-2-agonist.
5) Wait 10 minutes and measure FEV1 and FVC again (3 measurements). Use best FEV1 after the use of bronchodilators to calculate any subsequent fall of the referred parameter.
6) Explain to patient how to get the sputum.
7) Perform nebulization with ultrasonic nebulizer with 9 ml 3% saline solution during 7 minutes.
8) After blowing the nose and washing the mouth with water, collect the sputum in an appropriate recipient.
9) Measure FEV1.
10) If a fall occurs in FEV1 lower than 10%, repeat items 8, 9 and 10, using 9 ml 4% saline solution during 7 minutes.
11) If FEV1 fall is lower than 10%, repeat items 8, 9 and 10, using 9 ml 5% saline solution.
12) If FEV1 falls between 10 and 20%, the concentration of saline solution is not increased. The procedures are repeated with the same concentration of hypertonic saline solution, up to three seven-minute inhalations (total 21 minutes), or a drop in FEV1 greater than 20%.
13) If FEV1 falls greater than 20% or uncomfortable symptoms occur, discontinue the inhalations and begin treatment with bronchodilators.
14) Send the material to the laboratory of clinical analysis within 30 minutes after collection.
15) Fill in the induced sputum examination control form.

Bronchoscopic Examination Technique

Bronchoscopy with bronchoalveolar lavage was performed using Olympus® instrument with 2.2 mm diameter. All broncofibroscopy exams were performed according to the following examination technique: [53] after a 12-hour fast, the patient received pre-examination orientation, with clarification on the technique and possible complications. It was then placed in dorsal position and received oxygen through nasal catheter, with 2 liter flow per minute. Then local anesthesia with lidocaine 4% gel was applied in the nostrils, and lidocaine 10% spray was applied in the oropharynx, followed by gargling and swallowing. The bronchofibroscope was introduced transnasally, preferably, and in case of difficulty, orally. The examination continued through anesthesia of the vocal cords with 2 ml of 1% lidocaine without vasoconstrictor, and verification of their mobility for phonation manoeuvres, after which tracheal carina anesthesia with 2 ml of 1% lidocaine without vasoconstrictor was performed. Bilateral inspection of the respiratory tree was carried out and anesthesia with 2 ml of 1% lidocaine without vasoconstrictor was applied, if necessary. At that point, there was a collection bottle change, followed by bronchoalveolar lavage, after introducing the bronchofibroscope in bronchial subsegment (where there was a greater change in the computerized tomography, or in the middle lobe or lingula, if the radiological examination was normal). Bronchoalveolar lavage was performed by instillation of 0.9%

saline in 20 ml aliquots, for five times, and aspiration to recover from 50 to 75 percent of the instilled volume. After this phase, the collection bottle was changed again. Upon completion of the material withdrawal procedures, an inspection was made and then the bronchofibroscope was removed.

Induced Sputum Processing

In the clinical analysis laboratory smears were made on glass slides, according to the following technique: [54] a small portion of definitely purulent or granular (in the case of not purulent samples) sputum was picked up through platinum loop and placed at one extremity of the glass slide. To eliminate the contamination of this material with saliva, the small amount of pus or granules was rubbed until the other extremity of the glass side, still with the help of platinum loop. This manoeuvre was carried out in order to retain the saliva in the path of the smear displacement. Thus, the small portion of purulent or granular sputum at the far end of displacement was free from saliva contamination. Saliva retained in the path of the glass slide was removed with the aid of filter paper. The portion of sputum, then free of contamination, was stretched and placed on the slide for staining.

Zihel-Neelsen stainings were performed to search for alcohol-acid resistant bacilli; fresh slide with potassium hydroxide, *Giemsa*, *Papanicolaou* and *Grocott-Gomori* staining for *Pneumocystis jiroveci* and other fungi, differential cytological analysis, search for parasites, and *Gram* bacterioscopy for pyogenic bacteria. Culture growth for alcohol-acid resistant bacilli (*Löwenstein-Jensen*) and fungi (*Sabouraud* agar), and quantitative culture for pyogenic bacteria (blood agar and *MacConkey* agar) were also performed. [55,56,57]

Acceptability Criteria for Sputum Sample

Sputum sample was considered satisfactory if there were less than 10 squamous epithelial cells and more than 25 leukocytes per field of great augmentation, and the presence of alveolar macrophages. [54,58] If the sample was considered unsatisfactory, that is, if not representative of the lower airways, the induction of sputum would be repeated within 48 hours of the initial procedure.

Bronchoalveolar Lavage Processing

The bronchoalveolar lavage was sent to clinical analysis laboratory within 30 minutes after the completion of bronchoscopy. In the clinical analysis laboratory, the sample of bronchoalveolar lavage was centrifuged for 10 minutes, at 2500 rpm, followed by preparation of six smear slides. The following analyses were performed: Zihel-Neelsen stainings to search for alcohol-acid resistant bacilli; fresh slide with potassium hydroxide, Giemsa, Papanicolaou, and Grocott-Gomori staining to search for Pneumocystis jiroveci and other fungi, differential cytological analysis, search for parasites; and Gram bacterioscopy for pyogenic bacteria. Culture growth for alcohol-acid resistant bacilli (Löwenstein-Jensen) and fungi (Sabouraud agar), and quantitative culture for pyogenic bacteria (blood agar and MacConkey agar) were also performed. [55,56,57]

Acceptability Criteria for Examination of Bronchoalveolar Lavage

The sample obtained by bronchoalveolar lavage was considered satisfactory if it presented ciliated cells, alveolar macrophages and 5 to 10 percent at most of epithelial cells. [32] If considered unsatisfactory, the collection would be repeated within 48 hours after the first procedure.

Diagnostic Criteria for Pulmonary Diseases

The following criteria were used:

1. Bacterial pneumonia: presence of a bacterial morphotype predominant in *Gram* staining and quantitative culture growth of 10^4 or greater cfu/ml in bronchoalveolar lavage sample. [13,14,30]
2. Pulmonary tuberculosis: positive culture for *Mycobacterium tuberculosis* in bronchoalveolar lavage sample. [13,14]
3. Non-tuberculosis micobacteriosis: positive culture in bronchoalveolar lavage sample. [13,14]
4. Pneumocistosis: identification of the agent in bronchoalveolar lavage sample.
5. Other fungal diseases: identification of the agent and/or culture isolation in bronchoalveolar lavage. [13,14,59]
6. Parasitic diseases: identification of the agent in bronchoalveolar lavage samples.

Other etiological agents requiring demonstration in histopathological samples for diagnosis were regarded as unidentified etiologic agent, both in bronchoalveolar lavage and in induced sputum.

The examination of induced sputum was considered truly positive when consistent with the final diagnosis though bronchoalveolar lavage in a particular patient. [59] The demonstration of pyogenic bacteria was considered significant when a bacterial morphotype predominant in *Gram* staining and culture showed a growth greater than or equal to 10^6 cfu/ml. [30]

Once the results were confirmed, at the end of the study 20% of the cases were randomly selected for review of the slides by the same examiner in order to estimate within-observer variability. The same material was analyzed by a second examiner to estimate between-observers variability. [60]

Statistical Analysis

Demographic, radiological and laboratory variables were summarized as percentage or mean. [61]

Sensitivity, specificity, positive predictive value, negative predictive value and accuracy of induced sputum were determined, taking the diagnosis reached through bronchoalveolar lavage as the gold standard, according to the established criteria. [62,63] Additionally, the identified etiologic agents were described.

Kappa index of agreement for within and between-observers variability was estimated. *Kappa* values greater than 0.6 were considered relevant. [60]

Results

The study included 547 patients, with a mean age of 34.9 years, 495 (90.5%) of the patients were caucasians, and 370 (67.6%) were male. Diseases that motivated the service are shown in Table 1.

Table 1. Diseases that motivated the service

Diseases	n	%
Neurological	161	29,4
Gastrointestinal	138	25,2
Pulmonar	89	16,3
Dermatologic	38	7,0
Genitourinary	16	2,9
Miscellaneous *	105	19,2
Total	**547**	**100**

*Reumatological, anti-retroviral intolerance, psychiatric, not well-defined affections, lymphoadenopathies and others.

Fifty-eight patients with lung diseases were included in the study. Thirty-one patients did not meet the criteria for inclusion, since they showed less than 7-day respiratory events. Four patients were excluded from the study for refusing to participate.

The study sample was then composed of 54 patients (n = 54).

Characteristics of the sample regarding gender, ethnic group, duration of symptoms and $CD4^+$ cell counts are described in Table 2.

All radiographs and computed tomography of chest and mediastinum were also examined. Interstitial pattern was the most observed alteration (44.4%), followed by alveolar standard (22.2%). The standard was considered mixed when there were associate components of interstitial and alveolar injury.

Table 2. Characteristics of participants

		n (%)
Age in years*	35.7	
Gender		
Male		43 (79.6)
Female		11 (20.4)
Race		
Caucasian		46 (85.2)
Non-Caucasian		8 (14.8)
Duration of symptoms in days*	23.9	
Lymphocyte CD4+ T-cell count (/mm^3)*	124.8	

* mean
n = 54

Table 3. Radiological presentation of 54 HIV-positive patients with pulmonary disease

Radiological presentation	n	%
Intersticial	24	44.4
Alveolar	12	22.2
Mix	11	20.4
Pleural effusion without parenchymal damage	2	3.7
Mediastinal adenomegaly without parenchymal damage	1	1.9
Normal	1	1.9
Nodules	1	1.9
Alveolar + Mediastinal adenomegaly	1	1.9
Interstitial + Pneumothorax	1	1.9
Total	**54**	**100**

Karnofsky index showed that the majority of the patients were between 80 and 90, as described in Table 4.

Table 4. Distribution of 54 HIV-positive patients with pulmonary disease according to the Karnofsky index

Karnofsky index	n	%
40	1	1.9
50	3	5.6
60	3	5.6
70	9	16.7
80	22	40.7
90	16	29.6
Total	**54**	**100**

The most frequent isolated symptom was dry cough (46.3%). The combination of dry cough and dyspnea, as well as dry cough and fever occurred in similar proportions. Only one patient was completely asymptomatic (Table 5).

Table 5. Syntomatology of 54 HIV-positive patients with pulmonary disease

Syntomatology	n	%
Dry cough	25	46.3
Productive cough	8	14.8
Dry cough + Dispnea	7	13.0
Dry cough + Fever	6	11.1
Dispnea	2	3.7
Thoracic pain	1	1.9
Dry cough + Fever + Dyspnea	1	1.9
Assyntomatic	1	1.9
Productive cough + Dyspnea	1	1.9
Dry cough + Hemoptisis	1	1.9
Dry cough + Fever + Thoracic pain	1	1.9
Total	54	100

Results of pulmonary function test show restrictive ventilatory disorders as the most frequent (Table 6).

Table 6. Distribution of 54 HIV-positive patients with pulmonary disease according to spyrometric test results

Result	n	%
Mild restrictive ventilatory disorder	15	27.8
Within normal limits	13	24.1
Severe restrictive ventilatory disorder	12	22.2
Unspecified ventilatory disorder	7	13.0
Moderate restrictive ventilatory disorder	5	9.3
Moderate obstructive ventilatory disorder with reduced FVC	2	3.7
Total	54	100

Pneumocystis jiroveci was the prevalent etiologic agent, followed by pyogenic bacteria. In 10 cases it was not possible to identify the causative agent. Identified agents and final diagnosis are described in Tables 7, 8, and 9.

Mycobacterium tuberculosis was isolated in seven cases only through culture growth; bacterioscopy exams resulted negative. In four cases, *Mycobacterium tuberculosis* was isolated only in induced sputum samples, with negative results of bronchoscopy from bronchoalveolar lavage. No complication in sputum induction and bronchoscopy was observed.

Table 7. Etiologic agents isolated from induced sputum among 54 HIV-positive patients with associate pulmonary disease

Etiologic agents	n	%
Pneumocystis jiroveci	16	40,0
Mycobacterium tuberculosis	9	22,5
Pseudomonas aeruginosa	3	7,5
Streptococcus viridans	3	7,5
Streptococcus pneumoniae	3	7,5
Klebsiella pneumoniae	2	5,0
Proteus vulgaris	1	2,5
Enterococcus sp.	1	2,5
Klebsiella oxytoca	1	2,5
Serratia liquefasciens	1	2,5
Total	40	100

Table 8. Etiologic agents isolated from LBA among 54 HIV-positive patients with associate pulmonary disease

Etiologic agents	n	%
Pneumocystis jiroveci	28	46,7
Mycobacterium tuberculosis	10	16,7
Streptococcus pneumoniae	6	10,0
Streptococcus viridans	4	6,7
Pseudomonas aeruginosa	3	5,0
Klebsiella pneumoniae	2	3,3
Salmonella sp.	1	1,7
Proteus vulgaris	1	1,7
Enterococcus sp.	1	1,7
Staphylococcus aureus	1	1,7
Cryptococcus neoformans var. grubii	1	1,7
Serratia liquefasciens	1	1,7
Total	59	100

Table 9. Diagnosis of pulmonary disease type in 54 HIV-positive patients

Final diagnosis	n	%
Pneumocistosis	14	25.9
Pneumocistosis + Pulmonary tuberculosis	7	13.0
Unidentified etiologic agent	10	18.5
Pneumonia due to *Streptococcus pneumoniae*	5	9.3
Pneumonia due to *Pseudomonas aeruginosa*	2	3.7
Pulmonar Tuberculosis	2	3.7
Pneumocistosis + Pneumonia due to *Streptococcus viridans*	2	3.7
Pneumonia due to *Salmonella sp.*	1	1.9

Table 9. Diagnosis of pulmonary disease type in 54 HIV-positive patients (Continued)

Final diagnosis	n	%
Pneumocistosis + Pneumonia due to *Streptococcus pneumoniae*	1	1.9
Pneumonia due to *Klebsiella pneumoniae*	1	1.9
Pneumonia due to *Proteus vulgaris*	1	1.9
Pneumocistosis + Pneumonia due to *Enterococcus sp.*	1	1.9
Pneumocistosis + Pneumonia due to *Pseudomonas aeruginosa*	1	1.9
Pneumocistosis + Pneumonia due to *Klebsiella pneumoniae*	1	1.9
Pneumocistose + Pulmonar tuberculosis + Pneumonia due to *Streptococcus viridans*	1	1.9
Pneumonia due to *Streptococcus viridans*	1	1.9
Pneumonia due to *Staphylococcus aureus*	1	1.9
Criptococosis *grubii*	1	1.9
Pneumonia due to *Serratia liquefasciens*	1	1.9
Total	**54**	**100**

Data for comparison of induced sputum, taking bronchoalveolar lavage as the gold standard, are described in Table 10.

Table 10. Yield of Induced sputum, taking bronchoalveolar lavage as the gold standard, among 54 HIV-positive patients with pulmonary disease

Induced sputum	**Positive LBA**	**Negative LBA**	Total
Positive	27	3	**30**
Negative	14	10	**24**
Total	**41**	**13**	**54**

Sensibility = 65.9%
Specificity = 76.9%
Positive Predictive Value = 90%
Negative Predictive Value = 41.6%
Accuracy = 68.5%

Table 11. Within-observer agreement

	Second positive observation	Second negative observation	Total
First positive observation	8	1	9
First negative observation	0	2	2
Total	8	3	11

Kappa = 0.7

Evaluating the correlation agreement within and between-observers, after randomly selecting 20% of cases (n = 11), a Kappa index of agreement = 0.7 was observed, which is considered good. Only one discordant result was found in each category studied. Tables 11 and 12 show figures of within and between-observer agreement.

Table 12. Between-observer agreement

	Second positive observer	Second negative observer	Total
First positive observer	8	1	9
First negative observer	0	2	2
Total	8	3	11

Kappa = 0.7

Discussion

The results of this study show that the analysis of induced sputum is a simple procedure, without significant adverse effects and with good diagnostic yield in human immunodeficiency virus-positive patients with infectious pulmonary disease, compared to BAL.

The difficulties for etiological diagnosis of lower airway infections are multiplied in immunocompromised patients. This broad range of agents to which the individual is particularly susceptible complicates the diagnosis based only on clinical and radiological findings. In addition, there is no single propedeutic method with the desirable diagnostic capacity. In designing the methodology of this study, the following factors, which will be commented below in reference to their positive and negative aspects, were taken into account.

Inclusion Criteria

The manifestations of AIDS in different age groups in both the symptoms of the syndrome itself, and the prevalence and clinical state of opportunistic infections, has led us to consider only subjects over 14 years, therefore, excluding children. With reference to pulmonary disorders, it is known that in this age group, there is a different distribution of adults in terms of etiological agents. [64] Although pneumonia caused by *Pneumocystis jiroveci* is shown as a frequent infection, lymphoproliferative diseases, such as lymphoid interstitial pneumonitis, account for many cases. [13,14] If these patients were included, the sample would be hardly homogeneous and little representative. In addition, the procedures used in the pediatric field have indications and specific techniques, requiring therefore to be earmarked for this age group.

The minimum time required for respiratory manifestations was 7 days. It is known that this group of patients is also susceptible to viral infections of the upper respiratory tract, which usually has a self-limited course, even in this category of patients. With this attitude the inclusion of invasive exams for patients that could have their symptoms resolved spontaneously were avoided and, consequently, limitation in the number of negative results, not because of the employed method failure, but because of disease absence in lower airways, or for not using viral detection methods.

Although the radiological changes are the rule, a large number of etiological agents can show respiratory symptoms, but without concomitant image changes. In pneumocistosis, where reticular or reticulonodular infiltrate is the typical finding, the percentage of chest radiograms without alterations may reach 10% of cases. [12] Higher indices of normal examinations are observed in histoplasmosis, in which this fact is reported in up to 35% of cases. [12] Pulmonary tuberculosis, which in immunocompetent patients may have no radiological events in only 1% of cases, in patients with AIDS may appear in 20% of cases. [20]

HIV-positive patients with abnormal chest radiograph and without associated pulmonary signs or symptoms have high incidence of infections, especially pulmonary tuberculosis and nontuberculous mycobacteriosis. High prevalence of treatable and transmissible diseases in this situation justifies an aggressive approach. Studying this particular group of patients, Gold and collaborators established the diagnosis of pulmonary tuberculosis in 26% of cases, and nontuberculous mycobacteria in 23% of the cases studied. [21]

Exclusion Criteria

Previous empirical treatment significantly reduces the yield of diagnostic techniques for detecting pathogens in HIV-positive patients. Studies show that the yield of diagnostic procedures in patients without previous treatment is higher (91%) compared with those whose empirical therapy was initiated before the diagnostic procedures (64%). [49]

Similarly, the use of prophylactic treatment for certain conditions also presents effect on the incidence of certain agents. [65] Mayer and collaborators studied the effect of the use of sulfamethoxazole associated with trimethoprim as prophylactic agent for pneumonia caused by *Pneumocystis jiroveci* in the incidence of bacterial pneumonia. They pointed out that there was lower incidence of pneumonia among patients receiving antimicrobial, attributing this result to its activity against the most common bacterial pathogens. [66] Excluding this group of patients increases the diagnosis chance of pneumonia by pyogenic bacteria, as well as pneumocistosis. On the other hand, it could have influenced the distribution of agents found in this study. As the primary purpose of this study is evaluating the performance of diagnostic techniques, and not the incidence of pulmonary infections, the option was excluding them by their direct influence on the performance of the adopted techniques.

Unlike invasive procedures, the induced sputum collection technique offers few contraindications. The most important of them is the fall in FEV1 during the examination, which, when the rate exceeds 20%, contraindicates the continuity of the procedure. [52] This possibility was minimized with the use of beta-2 agonist prior to the procedure. The monitoring of pulmonary function during induction also increases security and is imperative to detect abnormalities that prevent the technique conclusion. [67]

Clinical, Radiological and Laboratory Methods

Chest and mediastinal computed tomography was another procedure performed in all patients. Despite its high negative predictive value and greater accuracy in detecting pulmonary diseases, this imagetic technique has no routine indication. [7] Its diagnostic value lies in the identification of hidden disease, characterization of diffuse parenchymal disease, identification and characterization of mediastinal lymphadenomegaly, and mainly to guide the needle for transcutaneous pulmonary puncture and indicate the best place for transbronchial pulmonary biopsy. [12]

Induced Sputum Technique

This study used inhalation of hypertonic saline solution in fixed time and increasing concentrations (3%, 4% and 5%) via ultrasonic nebulizer.

There are various techniques for inducing sputum, and with the use of different solutions. The use of hypertonic saline solution causes airway irritation and leads to bronchial secretions; in addition, there is the effect of osmosis with transudation of water into airway lumen. [68] In pioneer work, Yue and colleagues studied several inhalation procedures for sputum production in patients with pulmonary tuberculosis. They performed inhalations with sulphur dioxide, pancreatic dornase, acetylcysteine, distilled water and 10% saline solution. They observed that the 10% saline solution was the best inhalant. [69] Induction techniques and inhalants used have changed over the years. Currently, induced sputum is widely used for evaluation of inflammation in bronchial asthma and chronic obstructive pulmonary disease, being comparable to the invasive methods in this field, such as pulmonary biopsies and bronchoalveolar lavage. [70] Basically, three ways to perform the technique are used today: [70,71]

1. progressively increasing inhaled saline solution concentration, from 3% to 5%;
2. use of constant concentration (3%), with fixed time of inhalation; and
3. use of constant concentrations with progressive increase in the time of inhalation.

Analysis could also be carried out using total expectorated sputum sample, or selecting the viscous part, which is treated with ditiotreitol. [72]

It is known that techniques used with different saline concentrations and varied time of inhalation do not produce difference in cellularity, and that the use of ultrasonic nebulizer increases collection success. [71]

Regarding the use of total sample or selected sample, it is known that both methods have the same ability to distinguish between healthy people and asthmatics. [72] Since this study deals with the evaluation of collection technique used in a population with prevalent pulmonary infections, we opt to use the selected portion of the sample, since it diminishes salivary contamination. [71] It should also be emphasized that mucolitic solution was not used. The action of this agent on the viability of pathogens is not known so far, and its use is justified only for the analysis of cellularity. Chuard and collaborators also warn that it is not totally impossible that hypertonic saline can change the viability of some pathogens. [68] If this effect exists, it can be inferred that negative samples in patients with certain etiological diagnoses may have suffered this bias. Additional studies should be conducted to prove or refute this hypothesis.

Process and Acceptability of Induced Sputum

The technique described by Petrillo was used for sputum processing, in which the sample is processed so as to eliminate salivary contamination and analyze only the portion of definitely purulent or granular sputum. [54]

It is known that the respiratory tree below the larynx is virtually barren, but on sputum samples this condition is altered by the contact of material with secretions of the upper airways. This is particularly problematic for analyzing the presence of pyogenic bacteria. The microorganisms present in the salivary material come mainly from the gums, dental plaque and palatine tonsils. [73] Therefore, the mitigation of contamination in the expectorated salivary material is highly desirable. The use of different techniques that aim to reduce this confusion factor can be made. Mechanical removal of the largest possible amount of saliva, as performed through the technique described by Petrillo, coupled with vigorous mouth cleansing and mobilization of nasopharyngeal secretions previous to the collection minimizes this problem. Another way to reduce this bias is the microscopic analysis of the sample. It is known that the key to "true" sputum is the presence of alveolar macrophages and small amount of epithelial cells. [58,74] Microscopy sensitivity increases with good quality samples and also when they are quickly sent to the laboratory. [16] The biggest criticism of sputum analysis, as a diagnostic method for pulmonary infections, is regarding this potential contamination. Such criticisms are not unfounded, since approximately 45% of samples sent to laboratories are widely contaminated with saliva. [68] Induction alone does not improve the quality of the material, having similar yield to spontaneous sputum when appropriate samples are selected. [68] This problem has been greatly minimized with the combination of mechanical removal techniques of the salivary material and microscopic selection of samples through the presence of alveolar macrophages, polymorphonuclear leukocytes and epithelial cells, used in this study.

Gold Standard

The task of diagnosing a disease is not a perfect process. Almost always one starts up the work with probabilities and not with certainty that the hypothesis is correct. Associated with uncertainty, one frequently works with clinical conditions for which there are no objective and clear criteria. [62,63]. The ideal diagnostic test is the one which, when positive, indicates with certainty the presence of disease, and if not, indicates the lack of it. [63] When studies are performed on diagnostic tests, some care should be taken for the results to come closer to correct. Despite this, many tests are not rigorously evaluated before their release in clinical practice, and others are banned from use by systematic flaws in the evaluation process. The first important point in the evaluation of diagnostic methods is that all included in the study should take the test being evaluated and the gold standard. Moreover, tests should be interpreted independently. [75,76] Generally, the challenge in this type of study is to find a gold standard as close as possible to the theoretical gold standard. [77] If an imperfect test is chosen as a comparison pattern, the new test could have many false-positive results. [62]

In infections of lower airways, this is a frequent problem, and in immunosupressed patients, it is multiplied. There is no consensus on diagnostic techniques that should be employed with this group of patients. Specific diagnostic criteria were constructed to each possible etiologic agent. If less rigid criteria were used, the technique efficiency might increase compared to the gold standard, a fact that will be discussed during the analysis of results.

Another problem to be resolved was the diagnosis through sputum analysis in cases of bacterial pneumonia. The biggest problem in the diagnosis of this condition is the differentiation between contamination and colonization or infection. [33] Quantitative culture is a useful technique capable of differentiating colonization from infection. [16,33] One can assign an etiologic role to microorganisms when found in high concentrations and a contaminant role to organisms found in low concentrations. [34] Some authors argue that, in immunosupressed patients, even low concentrations are sufficient to cause infection. Pirali and collaborators found acute pulmonary infection with concentrations of 10^4 or 10^5 cfu/ml in HIV-positive patients, as well as a clinical positive correlation with the concentration of bacteria present in the samples. [34] The presence of 10^4 cfu/ml in bronchoalveolar lavage and 10^6 cfu/ml in sputum samples was used as a cutoff point in this study. [30,32] Using the same cutoff point for diagnosing immunocompetent patients may have caused diagnostic loss in some patients, but the use of lower concentrations could increase the number of false-positive. As there is no consensus on this issue, we opted for the first alternative. The authors believe that if the infection depends on the virulence of the microorganism, inoculum size and defenses of the host, the latter being undermined, as it is the case of patients with AIDS, perhaps a smaller cutoff point could be adopted. Further studies are needed to evaluate this possibility.

Results

Of the 547 patients evaluated, the majority were male, Caucasian, with a mean age of 35 years. This sample is representative of the Brazilian epidemiological universe, where the largest number of cases occurs between 20 and 39 years of age, and there is a predominance of male over female in the number of cases. [2,78] Similar profile was found among those selected for the study, predominantly males, Caucasians, and average age of 35.7 years.

Pulmonary diseases were responsible for 16.3% of hospitalizations. These figures are below the figures reported by other authors. Suffredini and colleagues described that in 65% of patients infected with HIV, the pulmonary is the first clinical manifestation of the syndrome and that 80% of individuals develop pulmonary disorder in the course of the disease. [4] Stover and collaborators described 47% of pulmonary manifestations during four years of observation of HIV-positive patients. [6] The changes in the treatment of AIDS generated an impact on the frequency of opportunistic events, and the systematic use of primary and secondary prophylaxis, which caused a decrease in the frequency of infections. [7] A decrease in the number of pulmonary infections in need of bronchoscopy, and in the number of examinations performed in this group of patients after the introduction of combined antiretroviral therapy is reported. [9] These factors may have been responsible for the lower figure of pulmonary disease as a cause of hospitalization and, consequently, the sample size obtained from the study. Another factor that may have contributed to this fact is the ambulatory handling of these patients, whose viral load decreases, and the rates of $CD4^+$ cells increase with antiretroviral therapy. If there is a decrease in patient hospitalization for this reason, it also carries the results to that population studied, that is, to patients who require hospitalization for the handling of their condition. The transposition of the results to an outpatient population needs specific approach later. Furthermore, no patient was excluded by finding themselves in poor condition or with severe hypoxemia, which infers that the studied population was not of patients with greater severity than those outpatients. This assertion is supported by the fact that 40.7% of patients had Karnofsky index of 80, and 29.6% had Karnofsky index of 90. These indices reflect those patients who are symptomatic, but in outpatient treatment. [50] Only four patients were excluded from the study, by refusing to participate, which did not affect the representativeness of the sample.

The average of $CD4^+$ cell counts was 124.8/mm^3. $CD4^+$ cell counts below 200 cells/mm^3 put the patient on condition of susceptibility to virtually all pathogens capable of causing pulmonary disease. [7] Therefore, the sample was not selected for any specific pathogen, so that individuals could possibly contract any pulmonary infection. Moreover, a low $CD4^+$ cell count does not exclude the presence of a pulmonary infection that typically occurs with higher counts. [20] The degree of immunosupression also correlates with radiological appearance of certain infections, becoming less useful in the differential diagnosis when it is near or below 200 cells per mm^3. [20]

The most observed radiological alteration was the interstitial pattern (44.4%), followed by alveolar standard (22.2%). The combination of alveolar interstitial events occurred in 20.4% of cases. No radiological pattern is pathognomonic of any etiologic agent, although each agent presents a tendency to show in one or other pattern with greater frequency. [79] In addition, interstitial injuries have a very broad and unspecific differential diagnosis. [10] In a study of chest radiogram diagnostic accuracy in immunocompromised patients with severe pulmonary complications, Logan and collaborators reported 90% of correct etiologic diagnoses in a group of patients with AIDS. In that study, chest radiograms of patients with proven etiologic diagnosis that included several causes of immunosupression were reviewed. [80] Perhaps the small number of patients with AIDS in that study and almost all of them diagnosed with pneumocistosis may have influenced the result. In the group in which AIDS was not a cause of immunosupression, and had a wider range of etiologic diagnoses, the percentage of hits did not exceed 34%. [80] The typical pattern of radiological pneumocistosis is reticularis or reticulonodular, perihilar and/or bi-basal infiltrate that may progress to diffuse consolidation of airspace. On the other hand, bacterial infections have consolidation as a typical pattern, but can cross with nodules, focal infiltrates and pleural effusion. [12] The etiological agents more frequently described in this study were pyogenic bacteria and *Pneumocystis jiroveci* and they may be responsible for the distribution of radiological patterns found.

The single most frequent symptom was dry cough (46.3%), which was predominant in combination with other findings, such as dyspnea and fever. In this group of patients, sputum is often not produced spontaneously. [16] Productive cough was observed in only 9 patients (16.7%), corroborating earlier statement. Just as the radiological presentation, the clinical picture is also nonspecific, and the most frequent signs and symptoms are fever and dry cough. [16,24] A study of Weinberg and colleagues showed that clinical, laboratory and radiological data failed to distinguish pulmonary specific pathogens. [47] In a prospective study of community etiological pneumonia agents in patients with HIV infection, Rimland and colleagues also noted that the clinical symptoms can not distinguish between the different etiological agents. [81]

Pulmonary function tests have their utility in this group of patients to confirm the presence of pulmonary disease in respiratory symptoms with normal chest radiograms, to see the presence of diffuse disease in patients with focal infiltrates and to quantify the degree of pulmonary affection in diffuse lesions. [79] In this study, 24.1% of patients had spyrometric test within normal limits, being diagnosed disorder in the remaining patients. Restrictive pattern was the most observed, comprising 59.3% of cases. This predominance of restrictive standards is in line with the distribution of radiological findings described earlier.

Of the 54 patients studied, a final diagnosis was obtained in 44 (81.5%). In 13 patients, two final diagnoses were confirmed and 1 of them, three etiologies have been identified simultaneously. Similarly, Rimland and colleagues described 13% of patients with pneumonia and HIV infection with two etiologies and 2% of cases with three etiologies. [81] In 90 bronchofibroscopies in HIV-positive patients with respiratory symptoms and radiological changes, Jensen and colleagues found 24% of microorganism association. The same author emphasizes the fact that co-infection has prognostic significance, giving the patient a higher mortality in the short term. Of the associations observed, the higher mortality rate was described for those with pneumocistosis and bacterial pneumonia. [26] One of the most frequent associations found in this work was pneumocistosis and bacterial pneumonia (13%), highlighting the importance of correct etiologic diagnosis in relation to prognosis.

Fifty-nine etiological agents were isolated in accordance with the diagnostic criteria in 44 patients where a final diagnosis was reached. The most common agent was *Pneumocystis jiroveci*, followed by pyogenic bacteria. *Mycobacterium tuberculosis* was the third most common group. Prospectively studying etiological community pneumonia in HIV-positive patients, Rimland and collaborators have found *Pneumocystis jiroveci* in 36% of cases, and bacterial etiology in 27%. [81] Assessing opportunistic agents identified by bronchoalveolar lavage in 99 HIV-positive patients, Durand-Amat and colleagues also showed *Pneumocystis jiroveci* as the most common causative agent. [82] Brazilian studies have shown this agent has greater frequency in this particular population, but they do not show bacteria as frequent etiological agents. [47] Bacterial pneumonia was the most frequent diagnosis in HIV-positive patients, with 63% of cases in a study by Danés and collaborators, leaving pneumocistosis as the second most frequent cause of pulmonary disease. [83] It is known that the spectrum of opportunistic infections is different in industrialized and tropical countries, the latter with the largest occurrence of pulmonary tuberculosis and bacterial pneumonia. Treatment with combined antiretroviral therapy and the introduction of prophylactic regimes, mainly for *Pneumocystis jiroveci*, have changed the distribution of etiological agents. [8] Results described here still point out *Pneumocystis jiroveci* as the most frequent etiological agent, and in spite of considering prophylaxis for this agent a criterion for exclusion, no patient was excluded for that reason. One possibility would be that the isolation of this agent in some patients meant colonization and not infection, since histopathological test for diagnosis was not required. Investigating the frequency of colonization and infection in HIV-positive patients and HIV-negative, Nevez and collaborators have shown that *Pneumocystis* may colonize immunosuppressed patients that is not caused by HIV, but in HIV-positive patients with respiratory symptoms, this possibility is remote. [85] It should be considered, then, that the distribution of etiological agents only reflected the local prevalence of different microorganisms.

Streptococcus pneumoniae was the bacteria isolated more often (6 cases), followed by *Streptococcus viridans* (4 cases) and *Pseudomonas aeruginosa* (3 cases). *Streptococcus pneumoniae* is described as the most often isolated agent in HIV-positive patients with bacterial pneumonia. [16,58] *Streptococcus viridans* has been described as a non-pathogenic organism and is rarely seen as the causal agent of pneumonia. However, reports of pneumonia caused by this agent in patients without immunosuppression, associated with the fact that quantitative cultures with a cutoff point equal to that used for diagnosing immunocompetent patients have been used, allows us to take over this etiological diagnosis. [85,86] Perhaps this microorganism has not often been diagnosed as a causal agent of pulmonary disease by the simple fact that it responds satisfactorily well to antimicrobian treatment performed with other microorganisms. It should also be noted that the group studied here consists of immunocompromised patients, in which the presence of microorganisms above a certain concentration, associated with clinical and radiological manifestations, adequately meets the diagnostic criteria for this pathological condition. *Staphylococcus aureus* was diagnosed in only one patient. Levine and colleagues, reviewing 129 consecutive episodes of respiratory disease in HIV-positive patients, showed that the agent was pneumonia in 8, or 6.2% of cases. [87] A larger sample of bacterial pneumonia cases would be desirable to provide more reliable results on the incidence of various bacterial agents.

The importance of culture for the diagnosis of pulmonary tuberculosis was proven by the fact that in 7 of 10 cases diagnosed, the bacilloscopy was negative. Conde and colleagues have shown greater sensitivity to the culture in relation to bacterioscopy for the diagnosis of pulmonary tuberculosis. [42] Weldon-Linne and collaborators, analyzing samples obtained by bronchoscopy in patients with AIDS, also showed better performance of culture in relation to bacterioscopy. [88] These data become especially important to HIV-positive patients. It is known that cavity lesions are characteristically richer in bacilli than in non-cavity ones. [89] In immunocompromised patients, the presence of typical cavitation is infrequent and it rarely occurs with CD4 cell counts below $200/mm^3$. Therefore, in this category of patients, paucibacillary presentation of the disease is the rule, further reinforcing the need for assessment of respiratory samples through culture, under penalty of diagnosis loss in a treatable condition with good prognosis and, especially, with high risk of contagion.

Analyzing a diagnostic protocol in immunosuppressed patients, Danés and collaborators have shown that the bronchoalveolar lavage technique had the greatest sensitivity. [83]

When comparing sputum induced analysis with bronchoalveolar lavage, we compare anatomically equivalent samples and, theoretically, with the same diagnostic capacity with regard to different pathogens. If we analyze the three cases in which induced sputum was considered false positive, we observed that *Mycobacterium tuberculosis* was isolated in the sputum sample without concomitant isolation in samples obtained from bronchoscopy. If additional procedures were performed, such as transbronchial pulmonary biopsy, open pulmonary biopsy or transcutaneous pulmonary needle puncture, perhaps these cases deemed false positives would be real positives, which would increase the efficiency of the technique in question. Since the sputum culture of *Mycobacterium tuberculosis* is considered diagnostic for the condition, there would be no justification under ethical point of view to hold such additional procedures in these cases. So, this could have been a factor of falling efficacy in the technique. Conde and colleagues found no significant yield difference between induced sputum and bronchoalveolar lavage in the diagnosis of tuberculosis. [42] Some studies show superiority of sputum analysis over bronchoalveolar lavage for the diagnosis of pulmonary tuberculosis. [46,90] The demonstration of high induced sputum yield in the diagnosis of pulmonary tuberculosis is not new, with studies already carried out in 1966, demonstrating its superiority over gastric aspirate. [91,92] An alternative would be a repetition of bronchoscopy, however Barrio and colleagues showed that the repetition of bronchoscopy within 30 days of the first examination through persistent pulmonary infiltrate, despite treatment, has no therapeutic implications. [93] The clinical follow up in these cases could be a strategy to define retrospectively the outcome of the examination carried out, if false positive or not. This attempt was not made, and may, therefore, have acted as a factor of error in the test interpretation.

How to explain respiratory symptoms and radiological findings in this group of patients whose etiological diagnosis has not been achieved? As reported earlier, there is not an ideal test for diagnosing lower airway diseases, and diagnosis can be lost by the method own limitations. Another possibility is the fact that some non-infectious conditions have been responsible for the clinical state. [17] Other studies also show the loss of diagnosis, even when multiple strategies are used. Danés and collaborators reached a final diagnosis in 84% of 241 patients studied. [83] In 42% of patients no agent was identified in a study by Durand-

Amat and collaborators. [82] A definitive diagnosis was reached in 83% of 68 patients with AIDS undergoing bronchoscopy in a study by Heurlin and collaborators. [94] Additionally, techniques could have been used that clearly increase diagnosis yield, such as polymerase chain reaction and cultures for viral agents.

Lentino and collaborators alert to the fact that sputum culture for common bacteria in non-selected samples and in patients without objective evidence of pneumonia would not have utility. [95] This is true not only for bacterial agents. Sputum analysis in HIV-positive patients before clinically recognized illness is not useful and not effective. [96]

No complication was observed in sputum induction and all were effective. In a study on the effect of sputum induction in oxygen saturation and spyrometric values held by Leigh and collaborators, no patient or control had severe side effects which needed to stop the procedure. [37]

The analysis of within and between-observer agreement revealed a Kappa index of 0.7 for both, which is considered good. Therefore, results presented here can not be attributed to dissonant analysis.

Conclusion

The results of this study show that induced sputum is an effective technique for obtaining samples of the lower respiratory tract in this group of patients. It is particularly useful in populations in which spontaneous sputum production is infrequent, and where traditionally invasive procedures for its production were performed. The results clearly showed that the best single parameter of induced sputum in diagnosing pulmonary infections in HIV-positive patients was its positive predictive value. This, coupled with the other results, poses this diagnostic strategy as a promising technique in order to reduce the need for invasive procedures in an appreciable number of patients, and can be used as an initial step in the investigation of pulmonary diseases in this group, reserving invasive collection techniques for those patients with negative results in sputum tests or with no answer to the initial treatment. Moreover, as a technique of easy performance that requires no expensive equipment, induced sputum is revealed to be an alternative approach in the initial diagnosis in places where access to invasive methods is not feasible.

References

[1] Organização Mundial da Saúde. AIDS Epidemic Update: 2007.

[2] Brito AM, Castilho EA, Szwarcwald CL. AIDS e infecção pelo HIV no Brasil: uma epidemia multifacetada. *Rev Soc Bras Med Trop* 2001; 34:207-217.

[3] Davis L, Beck JM, Shellito J. Update: HIV infection and pulmonary host defenses. *Semin Respir Infect* 1993; 8:75-85.

[4] Suffredini AF, Masur H. Pulmonary dysfunction in patients infected with human immunodeficiency virus. In: Pennington JE, ed. *Respiratory infections: diagnosis and management*. 2nd ed. New York:Raven Press; 1988.p.241-263.

[5] Murray JF, Felton CP, Garay SM, Gottlieb MS, Hopewell PC, Stover DE, et al. Pulmonary complications of the acquired immunodeficiency syndrome. Report of a national heart, lung, and blood institute workshop. *N Engl J Med* 1984; 310:1682-1688.

[6] Stover DE, White DA, Romano PA, Gellene RA, Robson WA. Spectrum of pulmonary diseases associated with the acquired immune deficiency syndrome. *Am J Med* 1985; 78:429-437.

[7] Boiselle PM, Aviram G, Fishman JE. Update on lung disease in AIDS. *Semin Roentgnol* 2002; 37:54-71.

[8] Slotar D, Escalante P, Jones BE. Pulmonary manifestantions of HIV/AIDS in the tropics. *Clin Chest Med* 2002; 23:355-367.

[9] Taggart S, Breen R, Goldsack N, Sabin C, Johnson M, Lipman M. The changing pattern of bronchoscopy in an HIV-infected population. *Chest* 2002; 122:878-885.

[10] Haramati LB, Jenny-Avital ER. Approach to the diagnosis of pulmonary disease in patients infected with the human immunodeficiency virus. *J Thorac Imaging* 1998; 13:247-260.

[11] Stringer JR, Beard CB, Miller RF, Wakefield AE. A new name (*Pneumocystis jiroveci*) for *Pneumocystis* from humans. *Emerg Infect Dis* 2002; 8:891-896.

[12] Naidich DP, McGuiness G. Pulmonary manifestations of AIDS. CT and radiographic correlations. *Radiol Clin North Am* 1991; 29:999-1017.

[13] Murray JF, Mills J. Pulmonary infectious complications of human immunodeficiency virus infection (Part I). *Am Rev Respir Dis* 1990; 141:1356-1372.

[14] Murray JF, Mills J. Pulmonary infectious complications of human immunodeficiency virus infection (Part II). *Am Rev Respir Dis* 1990; 141:1582-1598.

[15] Barreto SM, Molinari JF. I Consenso brasileiro sobre pneumonias: pneumonias em portadores da Síndrome da Imunodeficiência Adquirida (SIDA/AIDS). *J Pneumol* 1998; 24:95-100.

[16] Baselski V, Mason K. Pneumonia in the immunocompromised host: the role of bronchoscopy and newer diagnostic techniques. *Sem Respir Infect* 2000; 15:144-161.

[17] White DA, Matthay RA. Noninfectious pulmonary complications of infection with the human immunodeficiency virus. Am Rev Respir Dis 1989; 140:1763-1787.

[18] Stevens DA. Diagnosis of fungal infections: current status. *J Antimicrob Chemother* 2002; 49:11-19.

[19] Kennedy CA, Goetz MB, Mathisen GE. Absolute CD4 lymphocyte counts and the risk of opportunistic pulmonary infection. *Rev Infect Dis* 1990; 12:561-562.

[20] Shah RM, Kaji AV, Ostrum BJ, Friedman AC. Interpretation of chest radiographs in AIDS patients: usefulness of lymphocyte counts. *Radiographics* 1997; 17:47-58.

[21] Gold JA, Rom WN, Harkin TJ. Significance of abnormal chest radiograph findings in patients with HIV-1 infection without respiratory symptoms. *Chest* 2002; 121:1471-1477.

[22] Pierce JR. Simultaneous lung infections in patients with acquired immunodeficiency syndrome. *Arch Intern Med* 1994; 154:342.

[23] McKenzie R, Travis WD, Dolan AS, Pittaluga S, Feuerstein IM, Shelhamer J, et al. The causes of death in patients with human immunodeficiency virus infection: a clinical and

pathologic study with emphasis on the role of pulmonary diseases. *Medicine* 1991; 70:326-343.

[24] Speich R. Diagnosis of pulmonary problems in HIV-infected patients. *Monaldi Arch Chest Dis* 1993; 48:221-232.

[25] Masur H, Shelhamer J. Empiric outpatient management of HIV-related pneumonia:economical or unwise? *Ann Intern Med* 1996; 124:451-453.

[26] Jensen BN, Gerstoft J, Skinhoj P. The prognosis in HIV-infected patients with pneumonia. Relation to microbiological diagnosis. *Dan Med Bull* 1991; 38:468-470.

[27] Smith PR. What diagnostic tests are needed for community-acquired pneumonia? *Med Clin North Am* 2001; 85:1381-1396.

[28] Santamauro JT, Mangino DA, Stover DE. The lung in the immunocompromised host: diagnostic methods. *Respiration* 1999; 66:481-490.

[29] Gundy KV, Boylen CT. Fiberoptic bronchoscopy. Indications, complications, contraindications. *Postgrad Med* 1988; 83:289-294.

[30] Skerret JS. Diagnostic testing for community-acquired pneumonia. *Clin Chest Med* 1999; 20:531-548.

[31] Yeager H. Tracheobronchial secretions. *Am J Med* 1971; 50:493-509.

[32] Baughman RP, Dohn MN. Immunocompromised host. In: Baughman RP, ed. *Bronchoalveolar lavage*. St. Louis: Mosby Year Book Inc; 1992. p. 41-63.

[33] Lode H, Schaberg T, Raffenberg M, Mauch H. Diagnostic problems in lower respiratory tract infections. *J Antimicrob Chemother* 1993; 32 Suppl A:29-37.

[34] Pirali F, Longo M, Gelmi M, Colombritta D, Ravizzola G, Pinsi G, et al. Diagnosis of bronchopulmonary infections by quantification of microflora. *Eur J Epidemiol* 1994; 10:703-706.

[35] Jones FL. Aerosol induction of sputum. A valuable aid in pulmonary diagnosis. *Postgrad Med* 1968; 43:100-104.

[36] Rubin BK. Physiology of airway mucus clearance. *Respir Care* 2002; 47:761-768.

[37] Leigh TR, Kirby K, Gazzard BG, Collins JV. Effect of sputum induction on arterial oxygen saturation and spirometry in HIV-infected patients. *Eur Respir J* 1994; 7:453-8.

[38] D'Ippolito R, Chetta A, Olivieri D. Role of induced sputum in intersticial lung disease. *Eur Respir J* 2000; 16:573-574.

[39] Cohn DL, Stover DE, O'Brien RF, Shelhamer JH, Raffin TA, Hopewell PC. Pulmonary complications of AIDS: advances in diagnosis and treatment. *Am Rev Respir Dis* 1988; 138:1051-1052.

[40] Pitchenik AE, Ganjei P, Torres A, Evans DA, Rubin E, Baier H. sputum examination for the diagnosis of *Pneumocystis carinii* pneumonia in the acquired immunodeficiency syndrome. *Am Rev Respir Dis* 1986; 133:226-229.

[41] Bigby TD, Margolskee D, Curtis JL, Michael PF, Sheppard D, Hadley WK, et al. The usefulness of induced sputum in the diagnosis of *Pneumocystis carinii* pneumonia in patients with the acquired immunodeficiency syndrome. *Am Rev Respir Dis* 1986; 133:515-518.

[42] Conde MB, Soares SL, Mello FC, Rezende VW, Almeida LL, Reingold AL, et al. Comparison of sputum induction with fiberoptic bronchoscopy in the diagnosis of

tuberculosis: experience at an acquired immune deficiency syndrome reference center in Rio de Janeiro, Brazil. *Am J Respir Crit Care Med* 2000; 162:2238-2240.

[43] Ng VL, Gartner I, Weymouth LA, Goodman CD, Hopewell PC, Hadley WK. The use of mucolysed induced sputum for the identification of pulmonary pathogens associated with human immunodeficiency virus infection. *Arch Pathol Lab Med* 1989; 113:488-493.

[44] Rolston KV, Rodriguez S, McRory L, Uribe-Botero G, Morice R, Mansell PW. Diagnostic value of induced sputum in patients with the acquired immunodeficiency syndrome. *Am J Med* 1988; 85:269.

[45] Miller RF, Kocjan G, Buckland J, Holton J, Malin A, Sample SJ. Sputum induction for the diagnosis of pulmonary disease in HIV positive patients. *J Infect* 1991; 23:5-15.

[46] Anderson C, Inhaber N, Menzies D. Comparison of sputum induction with fiber-optic bronchoscopy in the diagnosis of tuberculosis. *Am J Respir Crit Care Med* 1995; 152:1570-1574.

[47] Weinberg A, Duarte MIS. Respiratory complications in brazilian patients infected with human immunodeficiency virus. *Rev Inst Med Trop São Paulo* 1993; 35:129-139.

[48] Luce JM. Sputum induction in the acquired immunodeficiency syndrome. *Am Rev Respir Dis* 1986; 133:513-514.

[49] Gracia JD, Miravitlles M, Mayordomo C, Ferrer A, Alvarez A, Bravo C, et al. Empiric treatments impair the diagnostic yield of BAL in HIV-positive patients. *Chest* 1997; 111:1180-1186.

[50] Mendelson J. Principles of neoplasia. In: Harrison TR, ed. *Principles of internal medicine*. 2ª ed. New York: McGraw-Hill; 1991. p. 1576-1587.

[51] O'Dell MW, Lubeck DP, O'Driscoll P, Matsuno S. Validity of the Karnofsky performance status in an HIV-infected sample. *J Acquir Immune Defic Syndr Hum Retrovirol* 1995; 10:350-357.

[52] Efthimiadis A, Pizzichini E, Pizzichini MMM, Hargreave FE. *Sputum examination for indices of airway inflamation: laboratory procedures*. Canadian Thoracic Society 1997.

[53] Strausz J. Pulmonary endoscopy and biopsy techniques. *European Respiratory Society*, 1998.

[54] Petrillo VF. A relevância clínica na preparação artesanal do esfregaço do escarro (judiciosamente selecionado) na bacteriologia dessa secreção: estudo comparativo com o aspirado de punção pulmonar transcutânea [Dissertação de Mestrado]. Porto Alegre: Universidade Federal do Rio Grande do Sul, 1987.

[55] Marshall JR. *Manual de laboratório clínico – microbiologia*. 1ª ed. São Paulo: Santos Livraria Editora; 1995.

[56] Luna LG. *Manual of histologic staining methods the armed forces institute of pathology*. 3ª ed. New York:McGraw-Hill Book Co New York; 1968.

[57] Behmer OA, Tolosa EMC, Neto AGF. *Manual de técnicas para histologia normal e patológica*. 1ª ed. São Paulo: EDART; 1976.

[58] Cordero E, Pachon J, Rivero A, Giron-Gonzalez JA, Gomez-Mateos J, Merino MD, et al. Usefulness of sputum culture for diagnosis of bacterial pneumonia in HIV-infected patients. *Eur J Clin Microbiol Infect Dis* 2002; 21:362-367.

[59] Pisani RJ, Wright AJ. Clinical utility of bronchoalveolar lavage in immunocompromised hosts. *Mayo Clin Proc* 1992; 67:221-227.

[60] Pereira MG. Epidemiologia. Teoria e prática. Rio de Janeiro: Guanabara Koogan; 1995.

[61] Dawson-Saunders B, Trapp RG. *Basic and clinical biostatistics*. Connecticut: Appleton & Lange; 1990.

[62] Fletcher RH, Fletcher SW, Wagner EH. *Epidemiologia clínica. Bases científicas da conduta médica*. 2ª ed. Porto Alegre: Artes Médicas; 1989.

[63] Menezes AMB, Santos IS. Curso de epidemiologia básica para pneumologistas. 4ª parte – epidemiologia clínica. *J Pneumol* 1999; 25:321-326.

[64] Sprinz E, Finkelsztejn A. *Rotinas em HIV e AIDS*. Porto Alegre: ARTMED; 1999.

[65] Kovacs JA, Masur H. Prophylaxis against opportunistic infections in patients with human immunodeficiency virus infection. *N Engl J Med* 2000; 342:1416-1429.

[66] Mayer HB, Rose DN, Cohen S, Gurtman AC, Cheung TW, Szabo S. The effect of *Pneumocystis carinii* pneumonia prophylaxis regimens on the incidence of bacterial infections in HIV-infected patients. *AIDS* 1993; 8:75-85.

[67] Holz O, Kips J, Magnussen H. Update on sputum methodology. *Eur Respir J* 2000; 16:355-359.

[68] Chuard C, Fracheboud D, Regamey C. Effect of sputum induction by hypertonic saline on specimen quality. *Diagn Microbiol Infect Dis* 2001; 39:211-214.

[69] Yue WY, Cohen SS. Sputum induction by newer inhalation methods in patients with pulmonary tuberculosis. *Dis Chest* 1967; 51:614-620.

[70] Olivieri D, D'Ippolito R, Chetta A. Induced sputum: diagnostic value in intersticial lung disease. *Curr Opin Pulm Med* 2000; 6:411-414.

[71] Kips JC, Peleman RA, Pauwels RA. Methods of examining induced sputum: do differences matter? *Eur Respir J* 1998; 11:529-533.

[72] Spanevello A, Beghé B, Bianchi A, Migliori GB, Ambrosetti M, Neri M, et al. Comparison of two methods of processing induced sputum: selected versus entire sputum. *Am J Respir Crit Care Med* 1998; 157:665-668.

[73] Gordon DF, Jong BB. Indigenous flora from human saliva. *Applied Microbiology* 1968; 16:428-429.

[74] Epstein MRL. Constituents of sputum: a simple method. *Ann Intern Med* 1972; 77:259-265.

[75] Reid MC, Lachs MS, Feinstein AR. Use of methodological standars in diagnostic test research. *JAMA* 1995; 274:645-651.

[76] Sackett DL, Haynes RB. Evidence base for clinical diagnosis. The architecture of diagnostic research. *BMJ* 2002; 324:539-541.

[77] Knottnerus JA, Weel CV, Muris JWM. Evidence base of clinical diagnosis. Evaluation of diagnostic procedures. *BMJ* 2002; 324:477-480.

[78] Ministério da Saúde. *Saúde do Brasil*. Brasília: 2002.

[79] Vander Els NJ, Stover DE. Approach to the patient with pulmonary disease. *Clin Chest Med* 1996; 17:767-785.

[80] Logan PM, Primack SL, Staples C, Miller RR, Muller NL. Acute lung disease in the immunocompromised host. Diagnostic accuracy of chest radiograph. *Chest* 1995; 108:1283-1287.

[81] Rimland D, Navin TR, Lennox JL, Jernigan JA, Kaplan J, ErdmanJ, et al. Prospective study of etiologic agents of community-acquired pneumonia in patients with HIV infection. *AIDS* 2002; 16:85-95.

[82] Durand-Amat S, Zalcman G, Mazeron MC, Sarfati C, Beauvais B, Gerber F, et al. Opportunistic agents in bronchoalveolar lavage in 99 HIV seropositive patients. *Eur Respir J* 1990; 3:282-287.

[83] Danés C, González-Martín J, Pumarola T, Rañó A, Benito N, Torres A, et al. Pulmonary infiltrates in immunosupressed patients: analysis of a diagnostic protocol. *J Clin Microbiol* 2002; 40:2134-2140.

[84] Pratter MR, Irwin RS. Viridans streptococcal pulmonary parenchymal infections. *JAMA* 1980; 243:2515-2517.

[85] Nevez G, Raccurt C, Jounieax V, Dei-Cas E, Mazars E. Pneumocystosis versus pulmonary *Pneumocystis carinii* colonization in HIV-negative and HIV-positive patients. *AIDS* 1999; 13:535-536.

[86] Sarkar TK, Murarka RS, Gilardi GL. Primary *Streptococcus viridans* pneumonia. Chest 1989; 96:831-834.

[87] Levine SJ, White DA, Fels AOS. The incidence and significance of *Staphylococcus aureus* in respiratory cultures from patients infected with the human immunodeficiency virus. *Am Rev Respir Dis* 1990; 141:89-93.

[88] Weldon-Linne CM, Rhone DP, Bourassa R. Bronchoscopy specimens in adults with AIDS. Comparative yields of cytology, histology and culture for diagnosis of infectious agents. *Chest* 1990; 98:24-28.

[89] Moreira JS. Valorização do exame de escarro. In: Palombini BC, ed. *Doenças das vias aéreas. Uma visão clínica integradora (Viaerologia)*. Rio de Janeiro: Revinter; 2001. p. 187-190.

[90] Ahmed AJ, Geteley A, D'Alonzo G. Diagnosis of pulmonary tuberculosis complicating HIV infection: superiority of sputum smear over bronchoalveolar lavage. *South Med J* 1992; 85:444-445.

[91] Jones FL. The relative efficacy of spontaneous sputa, aerosol-induced sputa, and gastric aspirates in the bacteriologic diagnosis of pulmonary tuberculosis. *Dis Chest* 1966; 50:403-408.

[92] Madkour MT, Warraki SE. The use of aerosol-induced sputum for diagnosis of pulmonary tuberculosis in Egypt. *J Egypt Med Assoc* 1969; 52:518-523.

[93] Barrio JL, Harcup C, Baier HJ, Pitchenik AE. Value of repeat fiberoptic bronchoscopies and significance of nondiagnostic bronchoscopic results in patients with the acquired immunodeficiency syndrome. *Am Rev Respir Dis* 1987; 135:422-425.

[94] Heurlin N, Elvin K, Lidman C, Lidman K, Lundbergh P. Fiberoptic bronchoscopy and sputum examination for diagnosis of pulmonary disease in AIDS patients in Stockholm. *Scand J Infect Dis* 1990; 22:659-664.

[95] Lentino JR, Lucks DA. Nonvalue of sputum culture in the management of lower respiratory tract infections. *J Clin Microbiol* 1987; 25:758-762.

[96] Kvale PA, Hansen NI, Markowitz N, Rosen MJ, Jordan MC, Meiselman L, et al. Routine analysis of induced sputum is not an effective strategy for screening persons

infected with human immunodeficiency virus for *Mycobacterium tuberculosis* ou *Pneumocystis carinii*. *Clin Infect Dis* 1994; 19:410-416.

[Translated from Portuguese by Wilson Schuelter]

In: AIDS-Related Opportunistic Infections
Editor: Claudia D. Galanda

ISBN: 978-1-60692-144-9

Chapter II

Mycobacterium Avium-Intracellulare Infection during HIV Disease: Persisting Problems

Roberto Manfredi[1]
Department of Infectious Diseases, University of Bologna,
S. Orsola-Malpighi Hospital, Bologna, Italy

Abstract

Still in the era of potent, combined antiretroviral therapy, late recognition of HIV disease or lack of sufficient immune recovery pose HIV-infected patients at risk to develop opportunistic infections by atypical mycobacteria, which are environmental organisms commonly retrieved in soil and superficial waters. Among these microorganisms, the most frequent is represented by *Mycobacterium avium-intracellulare* (*Mycobacterium avium-intracellulare* complex, or MAC). Health care professionals who face HIV-infected patients should suspect disseminated mycobacterial disease when a deep immunodeficiency is present, as represented by a CD4+ lymphocyte count below 50-100 cells/μL, and often systemic, non-specific signs and symptoms, and associated non-specific laboratory abnormalities. Mycobacterial culture of peripheral blood is a reliable technique for diagnosing disseminated disease. A set of two cultures may identify over 95% of cases of *Mycobacterium avium-intracellulare* bacteremia. Microscopical examination (Ziehl-Nielsen stain and comparable techniques), and culture biopsies from other normally sterile body sites (i.e. bone marrow, lymph nodes, or liver), also may be useful to pose a diagnosis of AIDS-related mycobacterial disease. Among drugs active against atypical mycobacteria, besides some anti-tubercular compound, the rifampicin derivative rifabutin, and the novel fluoroquinolones, the availability of macrolides

1 Correspondence:Roberto Manfredi, MD, Associate Professor of Infectious Diseases, Universiy of Bologna, c/o Infectious Diseases, S. Orsola Hospital, Via Massarenti 11, I-40138 Bologna, Italy, Telephone: +39-051-6363355, Telefax: +39-051-343500, E-mail: Roberto.manfredi@unibo.it

greatly contributed to improve both prophylaxis and treatment outcome of disseminated mycobacteriosis complicating the course of AIDS. Although multiple questions remain about which regimens are optimal, general recommendations can be expressed on the ground of existing evidences. Treatment should begin with associated clarithromycin (or azithromycin), plus ethambutol and rifabutin (with the rifabutin dosing depending on other concomitant medications that might result in drug-drug interactions). A combined three-drug regimen is preferred for patients who cannot be prescribed an effective antiretroviral regimen immediately. Patients with a CD4+ lymphocyte count below 50 cells/μL who do not have clinical evidence of active mycobacterial disease, should receive a primary prophylaxis with either clarithromycin or azithromycin; the latter could be coadministered rifabutin. Anti-mycobacterial prophylaxis may be discontinued in patients without a history of recognized mycobacterial disease, whose CD4+ lymphocyte count remains above 100 cells/μL, for at least three months while on combined antiretroviral therapy. With regard to subjects on secondary antimycobacterial prophylaxis, in appears safe to discontinue it when a sustained CD4+ lymphocyte count exceeds at least 100 cells/μL for at least 3-6 consecutive months, during a concurrent, effective antiretroviral regimen.

Keywords: HIV disease, opportunistic infections, combined antiretroviral therapy, *Mycobacterium avium-intracellula*re, diagnosis, treatment, prophylaxis

Introduction

Mycobacterium avium-intracellulara complex (MAC) consists of several related species of mycobacteria that are ubiquitous in the environment (especially soil, dust, and superficial waters). MAC is an infrequent cause of human disease in individuals with normal immune defence. On the other hand, in deeply immunocompromised patients, such as those with advanced HIV infection and AIDS, MAC still represent common and serious opportunistic infections [1, 2]. Among HIV-infected subjects followed in the pre-antiretroviral therapy era, disseminated MAC has historically occurred especially when the CD4+ T-lymphocyte count dropped at values below 50 cells/μL [1, 2]. Colonization of the airways (and also the gastrointestinal tract) by MAC can occur without evident morbidity; however, MAC colonization of these sites points out that the relevant patients are at increased risk for developing disseminated MAC infection [3]. The potent, combination antiretroviral therapies (cART) introduced since mid-1996 (12 years go), have been associated with a significant reduction in AIDS-related mortality, days of hospitalization, and the incidence of novel or recurring opportunism, including MAC disease [4]. However, there have been numerous reports of atypical clinical presentations of MAC, just since the introduction of cART [5-10], so that differential diagnosis remains difficult still in the third millennium. The diagnosis can pose challenges to the clinician because isolation of these organisms is often difficult. In addition, both active disease and airway colonization occur in individuals with structural defects or previous or concurrent illnessess, adding further confusion for health caregivers. Furthermore, these organisms are frequently contaminants, leading to false-positive diagnoses in patients with other active diseases. The treatment of non-tuberculoius atypical mycobacterial infections is as difficult as establishing a correct diagnosis because therapy is often prolonged, difficult to tolerate, and frequently ineffective. Given these challenges, especially in the face of a progressive increase in the prevalence of this disease, clinicians should be familiar with these emerging disorders, whose incidence may increase among immunocompromised patients other than those with HIV/AIDS [1]. There is convincing evidence that an effective treatment of disseminated MAC infection improves both survival and quality of life of patients living with HIV infection and AIDS [11]. Whether MAC can be eradicated once disseminated infection has occurred is still uncertain, but some evidences suggest that secondary prophylaxis may be discontinued in patients who have had sustained immunologic recovery thanks to an effective cART [12-14]. The treatment regimen for disseminated MAC occurring during HIV infection, should include at least two active drugs, in order to ensure efficacy and prevent the emerging of microbial resistance. The most efficacious drugs for MAC treatment are the newer macrolide antibiotics, represented by clarithromycin and azithromycin [15-17]. The preferred treatment regimen should include one of these last two macrolides, together with ethambutol and/or rifabutin (a rifampicin derivative with improved activity against MAC) [18-21]. Clarithromycin, azithromycin, or rifabutin should be administered as a primary or secondary prophylaxis to prevent MAC disease or MAC relapse in all HIV-infected patients with a CD4+ lymphocyte count persistingly under 50 cells/μL, despite cART co-administration [22-25].

Microbiological and Epidemiological Notes

The group of MAC organisms consists of *M. avium-intracellulare*, and other species of *Mycobacterium* that have not been classified in particular. In the past, it was difficult to distinguish *M. avium* from *M. intracellulare*, as the laboratory assay relied on organism serotyping. Therefore, it was common to refer to them as *M avium-intracellulare*. Of the 28 known seroagglutination MAC types, types 1 to 6, types 8 to 11, and type 21 are classified as *M. avium*; type 7, types 12 to 20, and type 25 are classified as *M. intracellulare*; while types 22 to 24 and types 26 to 28 have not been classified until now [26]. Using DNA probe techniques, it is now possible to rapidly identify *M. avium* and *M. intracellulare* [27]. However, in most cases of AIDS-related disease, disseminated MAC infection is caused by *M. avium* species, and from a therapeutic and prophylactic point of view there is no significant difference. MAC strains may vary in their intrinsic pathogenicity, which may explain why *M. avium* serotypes 4 and 8 are the most common organisms to infect immunocompromised patients suffering from AIDS [28, 29]. Some identified biological markers of the pathogenicity of the MAC organisms include the presence of plasmid, antibiotic susceptibility patterns, multilocus enzyme electrophoretic profiles, and restriction fragment length polymorphism patterns [30-32]. Superficial water, soil and dust have been implicated as possible environmental sources of MAC for HIV-infected patients (as well as for the general population). Duiring a documented nosocomial outbreak, the hospital water supply was the ascertained origin of a well defined MAC strain, with showed the same restriction fragment length polymorphism profile as that infecting a group of hospitalized AIDS persons with AIDS [33]. Furthermore, no apparent differences have been observed in the frequency of disseminated MAC infection according to age, gender, race, geographic areas, the different exposure to HIV infection transmission, antiretroviral therapy selection, and initial AIDS-defining conditions [34].

Pathogenesis and Pathologic Features

The mechanisms of spread and acquisition of disseminated MAC infection are still incompletely understood. As such, not all non-tuberculous mycobacterial isolates represent true infections, since they may be trivial colonization or contamination. Currenly available data support the hypothesis that MAC disease results from recent environmental transmission of MAC through either the respiratory tract or the gastroenteric tract, rather than from a reactivation of latent MAC infection. However, after acquiring a clinically-evident MAC infection, the eventual, underlying immunodeficiency becomes the most relevant factor which supports the eventual disease recurrences during the follow-up; it was true especially before the cART era, but it remains possible still 12 years after the introduction of cART. As anticipated, among HIV-infected patients with a primary disease manifestation, the occurrence of MAC dissemination does not vary among age groups [34]. Therefore, should reactivation of latent infection was the mechanism of acquisition, the incidence of dissemination would expected to increase with age, much like in tuberculosis (which is known to be primarily caused by reactivation of latent infection). From an immunological point of view, the risk of developing HIV-associated MAC infection is inversely related with the absolute CD4+ lymphocyte count. In one observational study, the measured one-year incidence of MAC bacteremia was 3% for patients with a CD4+ count in the 100-199 cells/μL range, as compared with 39% for patients with a CD4+ count under 10 cells/μL [2]. The same study also underlined that individuals with a far advanced HIV disease had a linear increase in the risk of developing MAC bacteremia over time, and the risk of developing disseminated MAC infection for patients surviving for 30 months after being diagnosed with AIDS was around 50% [2]. Other observational studies and prophylaxis trials added several, consistent findings: the risk of development of disseminated MAC disease ranged from 30% to 50% of patients with a CD4+ lymphocyte counts below 50 cells/μL, in the absence of specific antimicrobial prophylaxis [1, 23, 25]. In particular, the difficulty to mount a retrievable antibody response to MAC in HIV-infected patients with disseminated MAC infection may also suggests a recent primary infection, because deeply immunocompromised HIV-infected patients lack the ability to establish antibody responses to multiple, primary infections [35, 36]. Furthermore, literature reports of MAC colonization of the respiratory or gastroenteric tract preceding the occurrence of disseminated MAC infection suggest that the organism is first acquired from the environment and subsequently disseminated, when a severe underlying immunosuppression is of concern [3, 37]. Finally, the incidence of disseminated MAC disease among patients with AIDS substantially exceeds the frequency of MAC infection in the general population, as determined by population studies, and confirmed by MAC-specific skin testing, too [38]. As anticipated, MAC dissemination requires a susceptible host. By the year 1984, only 37 cases of disseminated MAC infection in non-HIV-infected humans were reported, the majority of them occurring in patients with identifiable, severe immunological deficiencies [39]. In the non-HIV-infected population, MAC infection generally cause localized lesions: cervical lymphadenitis in children, a slowly progressive fibrocavitary pulmonary disease in middle-aged men with a chronic, underlying lung disease (i.e. chronic obstructive pulmonary disease or COPD, lung emphysema, bronchiectasis, pulmonary fibrosis, and pneumoconiosis), or localized bronchiectasis in women who have a narrow anteroposterior chest diameter, pectus excavatum, scoliosis, or mitral valve prolapse and associated conditions (i.e. Marfan's syndrome) [40, 41]. The blunted immune response and the lack of local and systemic inflammatory reaction typical of patients with AIDS and a deep HIV-related immunodeficiency who develop disseminated MAC disease is consistent with the hypothesis that the key immunologic defects associated with dissemination are defective monocyte-macrophage killing of phagocytized MAC and a defective cytokine network response, including abnormally low levels of tumor necrosis factor (TNF), interferon-gamma, and interleukin-12 [42-46]. As a result of this extremely permissive immunological environment, MAC infection becomes widespread in extremely immunosuppressed HIV-infected patients, and it was the case of the majority of subjects suffering from MAC disease during the pre-cART era (i.e. before mid-nineties). In the majority of autopsy examinations performed in these patients who died of these opportunistic infections in the pre-cART era, MAC organisms have been isolated from lymph nodes, spleen, liver, lung, adrenal glands, gastrointestinal tract (colon), kidney, and bone marrow, but the multivisceral dissemination has virtually no limits, and may involve all body organs and sites. In fact, the magnitude of mycobacteremia has been estimated to be as high as 10,000 organisms/μL of blood, the equivalent of 10 billion organisms per gram of bone marrow, spleen, lymph node, and liver tissue obtained at necropsy examination [47]. Not surprisingly, the histopathologic examination of liver, spleen, bone marrow, or gut from patients with AIDS-related disseminated MAC disease shows a high-grade widespread infection, together with a lack (or a reduced) inflammatory infiltrate or tissue necrosis. In contrast, histopathologic examination of tissue from patients with AIDS who have localized, non-disseminated MAC infection demonstrates marked inflammatory reaction and tissue destruction similar to the histopathologic findings observed in association with non-HIV-associated MAC or mycobacterial lung or lymph node infection. On the other hand, at the time of cART availability, the rapid recovery of immune defences obtained thanks to the elevated and prompt antiviral activity of available anti-HIV compounds, is the basis of the so-called immune-reconstitution syndrome, which is more prominent just in patients with a prior-latent, or a recently acquired MAC infection (see below).

Clinical Presentation

As anticipated, disseminated non-tuberculous mycobacterial disease is not uncommon when advanced HIV infection is of concern. Prior to effective antiretroviral therapy (cART), nearly 40% of patients with CD4+ lymphocyte counts less than 10-50 cells/μL developed disseminated disease within one year of observation. The risk for disseminated MAC infection increases with progressively lower CD4+ lymphocyte counts. This AIDS-defining disease typically occurs when CD4+ lymphocyte counts are below 25 cells/μL, but patients with CD4+ counts less than 50-100 cells/μL are at elevated risk. Usually, a systemic illness caused by atypical mycobacteria (MAC) occurs as a severe, life-threatening opportunistic infection in patients with advanced HIV infection or AIDS, who has a CD4+ lymphocyte count under 50-100 cells/μL. Subjects who suffer from a disseminated MAC infection frequently show non-specific signs and symptoms, and multiple, but non-specific laboratory abnormalities. In many instances, a progressive worsening of constitutional symptoms may reflect a disseminated MAC infection, and this aspect can be incorrectly referred to the progression of HIV disease itself or multiple, HIV-related illnesses. Patients affected by MAC disease most commonly report persistent fever (not responding to a broad-spectrum empiric antibiotic therapy), remarkable night sweats, asthenia, extreme fatigue, anorexia, and weight loss up to cachexia (the so-called wasting syndrome). Aspecific abdominal pain or irregular-chronic diarrhea, may result from the involvement of retroperitoneal lymph nodes or gastroenteric mucosa, respectively, by disseminated MAC disease A notable hepatosplenomegaly and a diffuse lymphadenopathy, may also complete the clinical picture. Intraabdominal lymphadenopathy is frequent, as demonstrated using abdominal computed tomography (CT) in 14 of 17 patients with disseminated MAC infection [48], and may be easily detected by abdominal ultrasonographic studies. From a laboratory point of view, pancytopenia (represented by slowly progressing anemia, leukopenia, and thrombocytopenia), is the most common occurrence, while elevated serum alkaline phosphatase and lactic dehydrogenase levels, or low albumin levels have been also reported frequently. In a prospective, observational survey of MAC bacteremia conducted at a single-centre United States Hospital during the pre-cART era, the authors interviewed patients with a CD4+ lymphocyte count lower than 50 cells/μL regarding signs and symptoms, and evaluated the laboratory workup conducted as part of the diagnostic evaluation for disseminated MAC infection [49]. A history of fever lasting for more than one month, a hematocrit under 30%, or serum albumin levels below 3.0 g/dL, proved affordable predictors of MAC bacteremia. On the other hand, severe fatigue, diarrhea, weight loss, neutropenia, and thrombocytopenia did not seem to play a significant role in discriminating between patients who were subsequently found to have MAC-positive blood cultures, and those who were culture-negative for MAC, in an univariate analysis [49]. More unusual manifestations of viceral MAC infection include a broad spectrum of organic-systemic localizations, including oral (palatal and gingival) ulcerations, septic arthritis, osteomyelitis, endophthalmitis, pericarditis, and massive gastrointestinal bleeding [50-54]. Non-tuberculous mycobacterial pulmonary localization is almost always associated with symptoms such as chronic or recurring cough, sputum production, and exertional dyspnea. Hemoptysis, although uncommon, can occur (thus entering a frank tuberculosis in the differential diagnosis). However, also in these patients with a suspected respiratory localization, constitutional symptoms such as fever, fatigue, malaise, night sweats, and weight loss occur, and often predominate.

Diagnosis and Microbiological Workup

The diagnosis of disseminated MAC disease frequently poses severe challenges to the clinicians. As stated, MAC are ubiquitous to the environment and may represent contamination rather than actual isolates. Additionally, MAC and other non-tuberculous mycobacteria may colonize the airways of individuals with structural lung abnormalities, or chronic respiratory disorders. As a consequence, recovery of these microorganisms may represent airway colonization, rather than true infection. Therefore, discovery of MAC does not necessarily reflect disease. The diagnosis must be based on a high clinical suspicion that is compatible with symptoms and clinical features. When a respiratory localization is suspected, sputum cultures are not reliable since they are often negative, and bronchoscopic washing (or preferably bronchoalveolar lavage) may be a more useful diagnostic tool. However, in the right clinical setting, a single positive culture from bronchoscopic washing or bronchoalveolar lavage may be considered diagnostic. Tissue specimens obtained from biopsy stiudies (transbronchial lung biopsy, surgical lung biopsy, or excisional biopsy from infected tissues), are also diagnostic if they lead to the isolation of MAC organisms or show granulomatous inflammation on histopathologic examination. In the right clinical setting with highly suspicious clinical and imaging findings, tests in which cultures are negative should be repeated, as isolation of atypical mycobacterios is often difficult. Finally, a true *M. tuberculosis* disease must be excluded in all cases of suspected MAC, especially when pulmonary infiltrates and acid-fast bacillus smear positivity are of concern. With regard to patients with advanced HIV infection, systematic culture search of MAC from peripheral blood is a sensitive and easy method for diagnosing disseminated MAC infection. Mycobacterial blood cultures allow to establish the diagnosis of disseminated MAC disease with a very elevated sensitivity (ranging from 86% to 98% of cases in which disseminated MAC infection was subsequently confirmed at necropsy examination) [55, 56]. While one single blood culture set leads to identify around 90% of HIV-infected patients with MAC bacteremia, the adjunct of a second blood culture increases the identification rate up to 98% [57, 58]. The preferred culture assays are preceded by a lysis of peripheral blood leukocytes, to release intracellular mycobacteria, followed by seeding onto solid media (usually the classic Lowenstein-Jensen agar, or similar mediums), or into radiometric broths of commerce [59, 60]. Using this last radiometric assays, atypical mycobacteria can be detected from blood cultures in as few as 6-12 days, whereas 15-40 days are required with the traditional, solid media. Furthermore, currently available DNA probes and PCR assays can identify and distinguish among MAC species within as few as a two-three hours, after that a sufficient mycobacterial growth has occurred in radiometric broth or on solid media [27, 61]. As known, tissue biopsies obtained from normally sterile body sites also can prove diagnostic. For exemple, simple stains of biopsy specimens obtained from bone marrow, lymph nodes, or liver, may easily demonstrate acid-fast bacilli or a tubercular-like granulomatous lesion, sometimes weeks before positive blood culture results become evident [62, 63]. It is also possible that culture of bone marrow, lymph node, or liver, could be more sensitive compared with blood cultures, especially when a subacute-chronic disease has been already established, and a deep immunodeficiency concurs, as is the case of advanced HIV disease.

Therapeutic Management of MAC Infection In the Setting of HIV Disease

The treatment of disseminated MAC disease is seldom straightforward, especially in the field of HIV infection and AIDS. Diagnostic uncertainty is common, prolonged durations of therapy are frequently needed, and eradication is unlikely whilst underlying immunodeficiency remains present. Moreover, treatment regimens are expensive, and are often poorly tolerated because of frequent side effects, and the expected drug-drug interaction with multiple compounds frequently co-administered to patient living with HIV disease [1]. In some cases, patients with disseminated MAC describe the treatment as being worse than the disease itself. As known, mycobacterial organisms other than tuberculosis (and MAC in particular) are not killed by standard antituberculous drugs except ethambutol (at *in vivo* achievable plasma concentrations). However, based on extensive observational *in vitro* testings, at least 50% of MAC strains can be inhibited by achievable serum levels of a series of antimicrobial drugs, including rifabutin, rifampin, clofazimine, cycloserine, amikacin, ethionamide, azithromycin, clarithromycin, ciprofloxacin, sparfloxacin, and moxifloxacin. Unfortunately, plasma drug levels needed to obtain a complete *in vitro* killing of MAC (the so-called minimum bactericidal concentration, or MBC value) range from 8 to over 32 times compared with minimum inhibitory levels (minimum inhibitor concentration, or MIC value) [64]. While associated antimycobacterial agents have shown *in vitro* inhibitory synergism, a truly bactericidal synergism has been more difficult to be demonstrated [64, 65]. Moreover, in order to ensure *in vivo* bactericidal acitvity, the relevant drugs must penetrate mononuclear cells (especially macrophages) at a suitable concentrations, and must ensure levels capable to pass the bacterial cell wall of MAC organisms. Anyway, some reliable animal models of disseminated MAC infection showed that both single and combination antimycobacterial regimens led to reduced mycobacterial colony counts by several logs, and also improved animal survival [66, 67]. Medical therapy for disseminated MAC disease involves multiple agents, in order to facilitate clearance of organisms, and to minimize the emergence of drug resistance. The cornerstone agents include macrolides, ethambutol, and the rifamycin derivative rifabutin [1]. Three-drug regimens are preferred because of concerns for the development of macrolide resistance. In fact, some last-generation macrolides, in particular clarithromycin and azithromycin, showed very encouraging *in vitro* and *in vivo* efficacy against MAC. A multicenter, randomized, placebo-controlled trial performed in the pre-cART era, assessed clarithromycin monotherapy, in dosages of 500, 1,000, and 2,000 mg (twice daily), in patients with a primary diagnosis of disseminated MAC. The investigators reported a median decrease of over 2 logs in bacterial colony-forming units from blood culture specimens, thus demonstrating a more potent microbiologic effect than had been reported in earlier treatment trials, together with an affordable *in vivo* response [15]. However, a dose-response effect was not observed, but elevated gastrointestinal intolerance occurred with the 2,000-mg twice daily dosage. Although the 1,000-mg twice-daily dosage led to a greater microbiologic response *versus* the 500-mg twice-daily dosing, there was a trend towards an increased mortality in association with the 1,000-mg dosage [15]. When considering that monotherapy regimens were challenged, it was not surprising that drug resistance emerged after 2-3 months of isolated macrolide administration in this trial, affecting around 50% of patients, regardless of used dosages. Daily therapy is strongly recommended in the majority of cases. However, for patients who cannot tolerate daily therapy or those who do not require an aggressive treatment strategy, intermittent (three times-weekly) therapy, may be adequate. As anticipated, macrolides are the most effective agents against NTMB. As such, current guidelines recommend that macrolides be part of all regimens for NTMB infections [1]. Although effective, these agents should not be used as monotherapy to help prevent the risk of resistance. As a consequence, despite a growing evidence that the optimal agent for disseminated MAC therapy may be represented by clarithromycin or azithromycin, the macrolide administration should be "protected", after the combination with other antimycobacterial agents, in order to prevent or at least delay the emergence of microbial resistance, which is parallely associated with clinical deterioration, and a less favorable clinical outcome. A subsequent study confirmed that the 1,000-mg twice-daily dosage of clarithromycin has an adverse effect on survival compared with the 500 mg twice-daily dosing [68]. As anticipated, azithromycin is another macrolide which is fully effective for MAC treatment. In a trial of azithromycin monotherapy, patients with newly diagnosed positive MAC blood cultures received randomized administration of 1 of 2 doses of azithromycin, 600 or 1,200 mg daily. After six weeks, approximately one half of blood cultures were sterile in both groups, with a mean reduction in mycobacteremia of 2 and 1.55 logs, respectively [16]. As a consequence, we can suppose that the antimycobacterial activity of azitrhomycin was similar to that obtained with clarithromycin monotherapy. As already observed with clarithromycin, the higher dosage of azithromycin was related to a higher rate of gastrointestinal intolerance. A number of other antimycobacterial agents has been assessed in several randomized, controlled trials. In one trial performed before the introduction of cART, investigators compared the microbiologic efficacy of four-week monotherapy regimens of rifampin, ethambutol, or clofazimine in patients with previously untreated disseminated MAC [68]: only ethambutol achieved a statistically significant reduction in blood MAC colony-forming units, suggesting that ethambutol might be the most potent of these three compared antimycobacterial agents. A rifampicin derivative, named rifabutin, had been specifically developed for the management of disseminated MAC infection in the immunocompromised patient. In an early (1994) randomized, placebo-controlled trial in which patients with newly diagnosed disseminated MAC disease were blindly assigned to receive clofazimine/ethambutol or clofazimine/ethambutol/rifabutin (at 600 mg/day), approximately half of the patients receiving the rifabutin-containing regimen had a >2 log decrease in blood MAC colony-forming units, or sterilization of the blood, compared with none of those receiving only clofazimine/ethambutol combination [19]. The long-term clinical outcome of combination regimens including both macrolide and non-macrolide agents for treatment of disseminated HIV-associated MAC disease, was confirmed in a randomized multicenter trial published in the year 1996 [11]. This study included 187 patients with ascertained MAC mycobacteremia, who were randomized to receive clarithromycin at 1,000 mg twice daily, rifabutin 300-600 mg once daily, and ethambutol 15 mg/kg/day, or a regimen of ciprofloxacin 750 mg twice daily, rifampin 600 mg once daily, clofazimine 100 mg once daily, and ethambutol 15 mg/kg/day [11] The *in vivo* quantitative antimycobacterial efficacy tested significantly better with the macrolide-containing regimen, as was median patients' survival (8.6 *versus* 5.2 months; $p<.001$). Although multiple investigations contributed with the evidence of positive results, the composition of the optimal treatment regimen for disseminated MAC in patients with HIV disease is still uncertain. Based on the available microbiological and clinical data, a macrolide drug (either clarithromycin or azithromycin), should be part of the regimen. No significant differences in mortality rates was noticed in a randomized, double-blind trial comparing azithromycin at 600 mg once daily with clarithromycin 500 mg orally twice a day, in an ethambutol-based regimen [17]. Evidences coming from a 1995 trial of several clarithromycin-containing regimens suggested that clofazimine compared poorly with ethambutol as a second drug added to clarithromycin [18]. Furthermore, a randomized clinical trial that added clofazimine to clarithromycin plus rifabutin found a greater mortality rate in the clofazimine-containing arm (62% with clofazimine *versus* 38% without clofazimine; $p=.012$) [70]. Another randomized trial which assessed a four-drug, oral antimycobacterial regimen with or without parenteral amikacin showed no clinical benefit associated with amikacin adjunct [71]. A large, open-label, prospective, randomized trial comparing the efficacy and safety of clarithromycin plus ethambutol, rifabutin, or both for the treatment of disseminated MAC was conducted in the year 2003 [20]. Of 203 enrolled patients, 53 received clarithromycin and ethambutol, 50 received clarithromycin and rifabutin, and 57 received all three drugs. A complete microbiologic response (as defined by sterile blood cultures obtained at 12 weeks), was found in 40%, 42%, and 51% of cases, respectively. Notably, a significant improvement in survival was observed in the three-drug arm [20]. Anyway, another randomized, placebo-controlled study which assessed the addition of rifabutin to a regimen of clarithromycin and ethambutol failed in finding differences in the microbiologic response or survival benefit between the two stated arms [21]. Moreover, this last study detected a significant reduction in the development of clarithromycin resistance in the arm containing three drugs (2% *versus* 14%), thus suggesting a possible benefit in the field of microbial resistance, too [21]. Macrolide resistance occurs and typically results from macrolide monotherapy, although the concomitant use of fluoroquinolones has been suggested as an adjunctive supporting cause. Regimens that do not include ethambutol are also associated with the development of drug resistance. Unfortunately, in cases of macrolide resistance, mortality occurs within one year in approximately one third of patients and, nearly half of patients will die within two years [1]. In the immunocompromised host, treatment should be continued for up to 12 months; negative sputum cultures should be obtained in pulmonary localizations. Therefore, the typical duration of treatment may range from 18 to 24 months, but it can be even longer for some individuals, whose immune recovery last longer. Also in the cART era, treatment failure and recurrences of disseminated MAC disease are somewhat common. Patients are considered to be a treatment failure if they have not shown clinical improvements after six months of appropriate treatment, or have not achieved negative sputum culture after 12 months of appropriate therapy (in the event of isolated respiratory tract disease). Treatment failure may be related to treatment non-compliance or intolerance, local anatomic defects (cavitation or bronchiectasis, when lung disease is of concern), or drug resistance (especially to macrolides, as discussed above). Relapses and re-infections are also common, and may not be necessarily related to a rising drug resistance, compared with the underlying patients' immunodeficiency. Treatment failures are unlikely to have a successful course of re-treatment, in the majority of cases. Therefore many authors advocate aggressive treatment initially. Surgical resection may be effective in patients with focal (especially pulmonary) MAC disease, and is considered curative for solitary pulmonary nodules caused by MAC infection.

Antimycobacterial Prophylaxis Guidelines

Since up to 40% of patients with advanced HIV disease are likely to develop disseminated MAC, it makes sense to develop a strategy for preventing this disease in patients at risk (the so-called *primary prophylaxis*). Few specific risk factors, other than a low CD4+ lymphocyte count, have been clearly defined until now. Therefore, any current prophylactic strategy must be applied to the entire population at risk, specifically, patients with HIV infection and a concurrent CD4+ lymphocyte count below 50 cells/μL. Results of combined analysis of two randomized, placebo-controlled trials of rifabutin prophylaxis carried out in the pre-cART era, which included more than 1000 patients with advanced HIV disease, showed that rifabutin at 300 mg/day reduced the incidence of mycobacteremia by around 50% [25]. Interestingly, patients who received rifabutin and subsequently developed mycobacteremia had blood MAC isolates that retained susceptibility to rifabutin. However, neither each single trial, nor their combined analysis, demonstrated that rifabutin significantly reduced mortality. Combined analysis of both trials revealed an increased incidence of fever, fatigue, anemia, elevated alkaline phosphatase levels, and hospitalizations in patients who received placebo compared with those who received rifabutin. Patients assigned to the placebo arm in these last trials, however, tended to have a lower absolute CD4+ cell count, which may have accounted for some of the greater morbidity [25]. A further placebo-controlled study provided the first evidence that MAC prophylaxis could improve survival of patients with late-stage HIV disease. Six hundred and 82 patients with advanced HIV disease were randomly assigned to receive either clarithromycin (500 mg) or placebo twice daily. During a median 10-month follow-up period, only 6% of clarithromycin-treated subjects developed mycobacteremia compared with 16% of placebo-assigned patients (p<.001) [23]. Notably, the median patients' survival time was significantly longer for clarithromycin-assigned patients than for placebo-assigned patients (8.6 *versus* 5.2 months; p=.001). Dose-limiting drug toxicity occurred in 8% of the clarithromycin group, and 6% of the placebo group [23]. A prior trial had already provided even more convincing evidence of the long-term benefit of clarithromycin prophylaxis for MAC in patients with very advanced HIV disease. A total of 1216 patients with a median absolute CD4+ lymphocyte count of 28 cells/μL were randomly assigned to receive rifabutin (300-450 mg/day), clarithromycin (500 mg twice daily), or a combination of these agents [22]. Median follow-up of patients enrolled in this trial was 589 days (over 19 months), longer than in any other MAC prophylaxis trial ever performed; overall survival was approximately 50%. At the conclusion of the trial, deaths in the respective groups were: clarithromycin, 42%; rifabutin, 43%; and the combination, 46% [22]. In an intent-to-treat analysis, only 9% of patients assigned to clarithromycin developed disseminated MAC, compared with 15% assigned to rifabutin ($p<.001$). The combination of clarithromycin and rifabutin did not act better than clarithromycin alone [22]. Data from previous natural history studies and placebo-controlled prophylaxis trials would predict, in this trial group, a 36% incidence of disseminated MAC at 19 months in the absence of any MAC chemoprophylaxis [22]. Therefore, based on these last evidences, long-term clarithromycin prophylaxis administered to 100 patients would be expected to prevent 27 cases of disseminated MAC over the median lifetime of the population at risk (36 expected disseminated MAC cases, minus 9 observed cases per 100 patients, assuming a median survival of 19 months). In a third, earlier macrolide prophylaxis trial, 693 patients with less than 100 CD4+ cells/μL were randomly assigned azithromycin (1200 mg once weekly), rifabutin (300 mg/day), or a combination of these drugs [24]. During the median follow-up time of 514 days, the incidence of disseminated MAC was significantly lower in the azithromycin group (13.9%) or the combination group (8.3%) when compared with that observed in subjects treated with rifabutin only (23.3%). Dose-limiting drug toxicity occurred in 13%, 23%, and 16% of the three stated patient groups, respectively [24]. Interestingly, the occurrence of macrolide-resistant MAC disease has been an infrequent event in the reported prophylaxis studies: only 2-3% of patients given clarithromycin and only 1% of patients given azithromycin suffered from an mycobacteremia with MAC isolates that became resistant to these drugs. In the year 2000, two randomized, controlled studies have compared azithromycin with placebo in patients with a CD4+ lymphocyte count increased to 100 cells/μL or more while on a potent cART treatment, and no prior history of disseminated MAC disease [3]. Specifically, in a study published by WM El-Sadr *et al.*, a total of 520 patients were enrolled with a median CD4+ count of 230 cells/μL at the time of entry. There were no cases of confirmed MAC in either the azithromycin arm or the placebo arm over a 12-month observation period [71]. In the other study conducted by JS Currier *et al.*, which enrolled 643 patients, only two episodes of MAC disease were observed among the 321 patients assigned to placebo, and no cases of MAC occurred among patients who remained on azithromycin, leading to an estimated incidence of 0.5 events per 100 person-years [72]. In both of these studies, the discontinuation of azithromycin prophylaxis was not found to increase the incidence of MAC disease significantly during a median of 12-16 months of follow-up, suggesting that it is safe to discontinue primary prophylaxis in those patients who achieved a significant CD4+ T-cell count recovery attributed to an effective cART regimen [72, 73]. With regard to *secondary prophylaxis* against MAC, in the earlist study evaluating the safety of discontinuing secondary prophylaxis for disseminated MAC, the investigators prospectively followed four patients with a known history of MAC disease. Antimycobacterial therapy was discontinued without evidence of recurrence after 8-13 months of follow-up [12]. Later, in a larger, prospective trial (JA Aberg, 2003), a total of 48 patients discontinued antimycobacterial therapy [13]. All patients had been on a macrolide-based regimen for at least 12 months, and on cART obtaining a CD4+ count of at least 100 cells/μL, sustained for at least 16 weeks. Of the 48 subjects, 47 remained free from MAC complications for a median of 77 weeks off therapy. One patient developed a localized MAC osteomyelitis 16 months after stopping secondary prophylaxis [13]. Concurrently, in a French retrospective study, three patients of 26 experienced a MAC relapse [14]: one of them was extremely immunocompromised (his CD4+ count was under 50 cells/μL at the time of relapse), and the other two individuals developed atypical bone infections, concurrently with a CD4+ lymphocyte count of 126 and 160 cells/μL, respectively [14]. In patients with increased CD4+ counts on cART, who develop atypical manifestations of MAC, it may be prudent to continue treatment for a prolonged period of 12-18 months, and then continue chronic suppressive therapy (secondary prophylaxis), for life. It is also critical to remember to re-start MAC prophylaxis if immunologic and/or virologic failure results in a decrease in the CD4 T-cell count. Presently, the absolute CD4 T-cell threshold indicating re-initiation is still debated, although the United States Public Health Service guidelines again recommend to consider a CD4+ lymphocyte count below 50 cells/μL, as a risk threshold to start antimicrobial prophylaxis. To conclude, in the cART era it appears sufficiently safe to discontinue antimycobacterial therapy in patients who have been successfully treated their underlying HIV infection, and achieved a sustained CD4+ T-lymphocyte count above 100 cells/μL for at least three months, and were previously treated with a macrolide-containing therapeutic regimen for at least 12 months.

Immune Reconstitution Inflammatory Sindrome (IRIS) and Atypical Mycobacteriosis

Presently, there is no unequivocal definition for the so-called "immune reconstitution inflammatory syndrome" (IRIS), and also the management strategies of this emerging condition are not uniformly agreed [74-77]. The IRIS syndrome tends to occur more frequently in individuals who are receiving cART for the first time (or after experiencing a prior therapeutic failure associated with a deep CD4+ lymphocyte depletion), and who experience a rapid decline in HIV viral load while on an effective cART [74, 77], associated with a concomitant, relevant gain in their CD4+ lymphocyte count. Although there have been some attempts to reach a better definition of IRIS based upon the entity of CD4+ cell increases and viral load reductions, the development or worsening of signs and symptoms soon after the initiation (or the re-start) of an effective HIV treatment (usually reported as early or paradoxical reactions), may also occur prior to the establishment of laboratory-based evidence of a quantitative "immune reconstitution", established on the ground of the absolute CD4+ cell count. Maybe, the most frequent and best described cases of IRIS have consisted of atypical manifestations just secondary to a latent-subclinical MAC disease in the setting of HIV infection treated successfully with cART [5]. This MAC-associated paradoxic clinical reaction produces an intense local inflammatory disorder against indolent MAC infections, in individuals given an effective cART, and experiencing an "explosive" and rapid increase of CD4+ lymphocyte count (and cell-mediated immunity as a whole). In the field of non-tuberculous mycobacteriosis, IRIS is manifested by painful suppurative lymphadenopathy, pulmonary infiltrates, and skin abscesses, usually associated with pleural and also abdominal effusion. A case report is briefly reported and depicted in **Figure 1**. As anticipated, IRIS has been reported more frequently among subjects who start or re-start a potent cART regimen in the setting of an acute or a latent opportunistic infection, occurring with an underlying, deep HIV-related cell-mediated immunodeficiency. From a management point of view, since IRIS usually results from actual growth of the opportunistic organism, a pathogen-specific therapy is always indicated. Antiinflammatory agents (usually non-steroideal antiinflammatory drugs, -NSAIDs-, buy also corticosteroids), may be of some benefit on individual basis, while it is still discussed whether a slightly delayed initiation of cART in patients which start a potent antimicrobial therapy for an AIDS-related opportunism may prevent or blunt the occurrence, the intensity, and the duration of IRIS signs and symptoms.

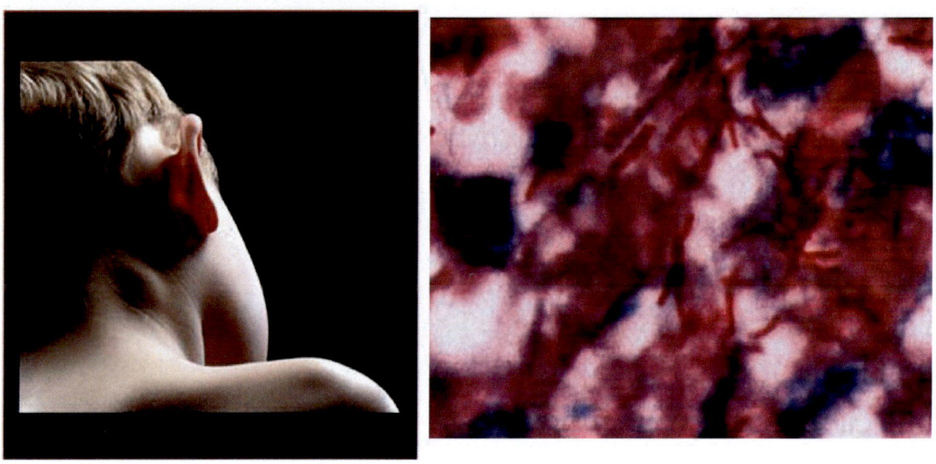

Figure 1. Immune reconstitution syndrome expressed by hyperpyrexia, fatigue, night sweats, bilateral pleural effusion, and multiple, enlarged lymph nodes, occurring in a HIV-infected patient who recovered over 200 CD4+ lymphocytes/μL after three weeks of a novel, effective cART regimen, started after failure and ascertained resistance to multiple, previous cART combinations. A lymph node biopsy disclosed a large amount of acid-fast bacilli, which were identified as *Mycobacterium avium* strains. Our patient already suffered from disseminated MAC disease, when 11 years before a diagnosis of full-blown AIDS was notified

References

[1] Chaisson RE, Moore RD, Richman DD, Keruly J, Creagh T. Incidence and natural history of Mycobacterium avium-complex infections in patients with advanced human immunodeficiency virus disease treated with zidovudine. The Zidovudine Epidemiology Study Group. *Am Rev Respir Dis* 1992; 146:285-9.

[2] Nightingale SD, Byrd LT, Southern PM, Jockusch JD, Cal SX, Wynne BA. Incidence of *Mycobacterium avium-intracellulare* complex bacteremia in human immunodeficiency virus-positive patients. *J Infect Dis* 1992; 165:1082-5.

[3] Chin DP, Hopewell PC, Yajko DM, et al. *Mycobacterium avium* complex in the respiratory or gastrointestinal tract and the risk of *M. avium* complex bacteremia in patients with human immunodeficiency virus infection. *J Infect Dis* 1994; 169:289-95.

[4] Palella FJ, Delaney KM, Moorman AC, et al. Declining morbidity and mortality among patients with advanced human immunodeficiency virus infection. HIV Outpatient Study Investigators. *N Engl J Med* 1998; 338:853-60.

[5] Phillips P, Kwiatkowski MB, Copland M, Craib K, Montaner J. Mycobacterial lymphadenitis associated with the initiation of combination antiretroviral therapy. *J Acquir Immune Defic Syndr Hum Retrovirol* 1999; 20:122-8.

[6] Sheppard DC, Sullam PM. Primary septic arthritis and osteomyelitis due to *Mycobacterium avium* complex in a patient with AIDS. *Clin Infect Dis* 1997; 25:925-6.

[7] Miller RS, Thomas SJ, Hospenthal DR, Oster CN. Isolated *Mycobacterium avium* complex osteomyelitis in a patient with AIDS. In: Program and Abstracts of the 35th Annual Meeting of the Infectious Diseases Society of America; September 13-16, 1997; San Francisco. Abstract 574.

[8] Alisky JM, Schlesinger L. Isolated cavitary pulmonary *Mycobacterium avium* complex infection in a patient with AIDS. *Clin Infect Dis* 1998; 27:1542-3.

[9] Hocqueloux L, Lesprit P, Herrmann JL, et al.. Pulmonary *Mycobacterium avium* complex disease without dissemination in HIV-infected patients. Chest 1998; 113:542-

[10] Race EM, Adelson-Mitty J, Kriegel GR, et al. Focal mycobacterial lymphadenitis following initiation of protease-inhibitor therapy in patients with advanced HIV-1 disease. *Lancet* 1998; 351:252-5.

[11] Shafran SD, Singer J, Zarowny DP, et al. A comparison of two regimens for the treatment of *Mycobacterium avium* complex bacteremia in AIDS: rifabutin, ethambutol, and clarithromycin *versus* rifampin, ethambutol, clofazimine, and ciprofloxacin. *N Engl J Med* 1996; 335:377-83.

[12] Aberg JA, Yajko DM, Jacobson MA. Eradication of AIDS-related disseminated *Mycobacterium avium* complex infection after 12 months of antimycobacterial therapy combined with highly active antiretroviral therapy. *J Infect Dis* 1998; 178:1446-9.

[13] Aberg JA, Williams PL, Liu T, et al. A study of discontinuing maintenance therapy in human immunodeficiency virus-infected subjects with disseminated *Mycobacterium avium* complex. *J Infect Dis* 2003; 187:1046-52.

[14] Zeller V, Truffot C, Agher R, et al. Discontinuation of secondary prophylaxis against disseminated Mycobacterium avium complex infection and toxoplasmic encephalitis. *Clin Infect Dis* 2002; 34:662-7.

[15] Chaisson RE, Benson CA, Dubé MP, et al. Clarithromycin therapy for bacteremic *Mycobacterium avium* complex disease. A randomized, double-blind, dose-ranging study in patients with AIDS. AIDS. *Ann Intern Med* 1994; 121:905-11.

[16] Koletar SL, Berry AJ, Cynamon MH, et al. Azithromycin as treatment for disseminated *Mycobacterium avium* complex in AIDS patients. *Antimicrob Agents Chemother* 1999; 43:2869-72.

[17] Dunne M, Fessel J, Kumar P, et al. A randomized, double-blind trial comparing azithromycin and clarithromycin in the treatment of disseminated *Mycobacterium avium* infection in patients with human immunodeficiency virus. *Clin Infect Dis* 2000; 31:1245-52.

[18] Dubé MP, Sattler FR, Torriani FJ, et al. A randomized evaluation of ethambutol for prevention of relapse and drug resistance during treatment of *Mycobacterium avium*

complex bacteremia with clarithromycin-based combination therapy. California Collaborative Treatment Group. *J Infect Dis* 1997; 176:1225-32.

[19] Sullam PM, Gordin FM, Wynne BA. Efficacy of rifabutin in the treatment of disseminated infection due to *Mycobacterium avium* complex. The Rifabutin Treatment Group. *Clin Infect Dis* 1994; 19:84-6.

[20] Benson CA, Williams PL, Currier JS, et al. A prospective, randomized trial examining the efficacy and safety of clarithromycin in combination with ethambutol, rifabutin, or both for the treatment of disseminated *Mycobacterium avium* complex disease in persons with acquired immunodeficiency syndrome. *Clin Infect Dis* 2003; 37:1234-43.

[21] Gordin FM, Sullam PM, Shafran SD, et al. A randomized, placebo-controlled study of rifabutin added to a regimen of clarithromycin and ethambutol for treatment of disseminated infection with *Mycobacterium avium* complex. Clin Infect Dis 1999; 28:1080-5.

[22] Benson CA, Williams PL, Cohn DL, et al. Clarithromycin or rifabutin alone or in combination for primary prophylaxis of *Mycobacterium avium* complex disease in patients with AIDS: A randomized, double-blind, placebo-controlled trial. *J Infect Dis* 2000; 181:1289-97.

[23] Pierce M, Crampton S, Henry D, et al. A randomized trial of clarithromycin as prophylaxis against disseminated Mycobacterium avium complex infection in patients with advanced acquired immunodeficiency syndrome. *N Engl J Med* 1996; 335:384-91.

[24] Havlir DV, Dube MP, Sattler FR, et al. Prophylaxis against disseminated *Mycobacterium avium* complex with weekly azithromycin, daily rifabutin, or both. *N Engl J Med* 1996; 335:392-8.

[25] Nightingale SD, Cameron DW, Gordin FM, et al. Two controlled trials of rifabutin prophylaxis against *Mycobacterium avium* complex infection in AIDS. *N Engl J Med* 1993; 329:828-33.

[26] Wolinsky E. Mycobacterial diseases other than tuberculosis. *Clin Infect Dis* 1992; 15:1-10.

[27] Kiehn TE, Edwards FF. Rapid identification using a specific DNA probe of *Mycobacterium avium* complex from patients with acquired immunodeficiency syndrome. *J Clin Microbiol* 1987; 25:1551-2.

[28] Yakrus MA, Good RC. Geographic distribution, frequency, and specimen source of *Mycobacterium avium* complex serotypes isolated from patients with acquired immunodeficiency syndrome. *J Clin Microbiol* 1990; 28:926-9.

[29] Tsang AY, Denner JC, Brennan PJ, McClatchy JK. Clinical and epidemiological importance of typing of Mycobacterium avium complex isolates. *J Clin Microbiol* 1992; 30:479-84.

[30] Crawford JT, Bates JH. Analysis of plasmids in *Mycobacterium avium-intracellulare* isolates from persons with acquired immunodeficiency syndrome. *Am Rev Respir Dis* 1986; 134:659-61.

[31] Horsburgh CR, Jr., Cohn DL, Roberts RB, et al. *Mycobacterium avium-M. intracellulare* isolates from patients with or without acquired immunodeficiency

syndrome. *Antimicrob Agents Chemother* 1986; 30:955-7.
[32] Hampson SJ, Portaels F, Thompson J, et al. DNA probes demonstrate a single highly conserved strain of Mycobacterium avium infecting AIDS patients. *Lancet* 1989; 1:65-8.
[33] von Reyn CF, Maslow JN, Barber TW, Falkinham JO, Arbeit RD. Persistent colonisation of potable water as a source of *Mycobacterium avium* infection in AIDS. *Lancet* 1994; 343:1137-41.
[34] Horsburgh CR, Jr., Selik RM. The epidemiology of disseminated nontuberculous mycobacterial infection in the acquired immunodeficiency syndrome (AIDS). *Am Rev Respir Dis* 1989; 139:4-7.
[35] Winter SM, Bernard EM, Gold JW, Armstrong D. Humoral response to disseminated infection by *Mycobacterium avium-Mycobacterium intracellulare* in acquired immunodeficiency syndrome and hairy cell leukemia. *J Infect Dis* 1985; 151:523-7.
[36] Wayne LG, Young LS, Bertram M. Absence of mycobacterial antibody in patients with acquired immune deficiency syndrome. *Eur J Clin Microbiol* 1986; 5:363-5.
[37] Jacobson MA, Hopewell PC, Yajko DM, et al. Natural history of disseminated *Mycobacterium avium* complex infection in AIDS. *J Infect Dis* 1991; 164:994-8.
[38] von Reyn CF, Barber TW, Arbeit RD, et al. Evidence of previous infection with *Mycobacterium avium-Mycobacterium intracellulare* complex among healthy subjects: an international study of dominant mycobacterial skin test reactions. *J Infect Dis* 1993; 168:1553-8.
[39] Horsburgh CR, Jr., Mason UG, 3rd, Farhi DC, Iseman MD. Disseminated infection with *Mycobacterium avium-intracellulare*. A report of 13 cases and a review of the literature. *Medicine (Baltimore)* 1985; 64:36-48.
[40] Wolinsky E. Nontuberculous mycobacteria and associated diseases. *Am Rev Respir Dis* 1979; 119:107-59.
[41] Iseman MD, Buschman DL, Ackerson LM. Pectus excavatum and scoliosis. Thoracic anomalies associated with pulmonary disease caused by Mycobacterium avium complex. *Am Rev Respir Dis* 1991; 144:914-6.
[42] Denis M, Gregg EO. Recombinant tumour necrosis factor-alpha decreases whereas recombinant interleukin-6 increases growth of a virulent strain of *Mycobacterium avium* in human macrophages. *Immunology* 1990; 71:139-41.
[43] Appelberg R, Castro AG, Pedrosa J, Silva RA, Orme IM, Minoprio P. Role of gamma interferon and tumor necrosis factor alpha during T-cell-independent and -dependent phases of *Mycobacterium avium* infection. *Infect Immun 1*994; 62:3962-71.
[44] Castro AG, Silva RA, Appelberg R. Endogenously produced IL-12 is required for the induction of protective T cells during *Mycobacterium avium* infections in mice. *J Immunol* 1995; 155:2013-9.
[45] Newman GW, Guarnaccia JR, Vance EA, Wu JY, Remold HG, Kazanjian PH. Interleukin-12 enhances antigen-specific proliferation of peripheral blood mononuclear cells from HIV-positive and negative donors in response to *Mycobacterium avium*. *AIDS* 1994; 8:1413-9.

[46] Zakowski P, Fligiel S, Berlin GW, Johnson L, Jr. Disseminated *Mycobacterium avium-intracellulare* infection in homosexual men dying of acquired immunodeficiency. *JAMA* 1982; 248:2980-2.

[47] Wong B, Edwards FF, Kiehn TE, et al. Continuous high-grade *Mycobacterium avium-intracellulare* bacteremia in patients with the acquired immune deficiency syndrome. *Am J Med* 1985; 78:35-40.

[48] Nyberg DA, Federle MP, Jeffrey RB, Bottles K, Wofsy CB. Abdominal CT findings of disseminated *Mycobacterium avium-intracellulare* in AIDS. *Am J Roentgenol* 1985; 145:297-9.

[49] Chin DP, Hopewell PC, Yajko DM, et al. *Mycobacterium avium* complex in the respiratory or gastrointestinal tract and the risk of *M. avium* complex bacteremia in patients with human immunodeficiency virus infection. *J Infect Dis* 1994; 169:289-95.

[50] Volpe F, Schwimmer A, Barr C. Oral manifestation of disseminated *Mycobacterium avium intracellulare* in a patient with AIDS. *Oral Surg Oral Med Oral Pathol* 1985; 60:567-70.

[51] Blumenthal DR, Zucker JR, Hawkins CC. *Mycobacterium avium* complex-induced septic arthritis and osteomyelitis in a patient with the acquired immunodeficiency syndrome. *Arthritis Rheum* 1990; 33:757-8.

[52] Cohen JI, Saragas SJ. Endophthalmitis due to *Mycobacterium avium* in a patient with AIDS. *Ann Ophthalmol* 1990; 22:47-51.

[53] Woods GL, Goldsmith JC. Fatal pericarditis due to *Mycobacterium avium-intracellulare* in acquired immunodeficiency syndrome. *Chest* 1989; 95:1355-7.

[54] Cappell MS, Gupta A. Gastrointestinal hemorrhage due to gastrointestinal *Mycobacterium avium intracellulare* or esophageal candidiasis in patients with the acquired immunodeficiency syndrome. Am J Gastroenterol 1992; 87:224-9.

[55] Hawkins CC, Gold JW, Whimbey E, et al. *Mycobacterium avium* complex infections in patients with the acquired immunodeficiency syndrome. *Ann Intern Med* 1986; 105:184-8.

[56] Wallace JM, Hannah JB. *Mycobacterium avium* complex infection in patients with the acquired immunodeficiency syndrome. A clinicopathologic study. *Chest* 1988; 93:926-32.

[57] Yagupsky P, Menegus MA. Cumulative positivity rates of multiple blood cultures for *Mycobacterium avium-intracellulare* and *Cryptococcus neoformans* in patients with the acquired immunodeficiency syndrome. *Arch Pathol Lab Med* 1990; 114:923-5.

[58] Reves R, Stone-Venohr B, Hildred G, et al. Utility of paired blood cultures in the diagnosis of disseminated Mycobacterium avium complex infection (abstract). In: Proceedings of the 8th International Conference on AIDS, Amsterdam, July 19-24, 1992. Amsterdam: Dutch Foundation 1992;127.

[59] Roberts GD, Koneman EW, Kin YK. Mycobacterium. In: Balows A, Hausler WJ Jr, Herrmann KL, et al., eds. Manual of Clinical Microbiology. Washington, DC: American Society of Microbiology, 1991;304-339.

[60] Shanson DC, Dryden MS. Comparison of methods for isolating *Mycobacterium avium-intracellulare* from blood of patients with AIDS. *J Clin Pathol* 1988; 41:687-90.

[61] Gazzola L, Zanini F, Zerbi P, Franzetti F, Gori A. The usefulness of PCR assay in

diagnosing disseminated mycobacterial infection in AIDS patients. *Eur J Clin Microbiol Infect Dis* 2008; 27:163-6.

[62] Nichols L, Florentine B, Lewis W, Sattler F, Rarick MU, Brynes RK. Bone marrow examination for the diagnosis of mycobacterial and fungal infections in the acquired immunodeficiency syndrome. *Arch Pathol Lab Med* 1991; 115:1125-32.

[63] Northfelt DW, Mayer A, Kaplan LD, et al. The usefulness of diagnostic bone marrow examination in patients with human immunodeficiency virus (HIV) infection. *J Acquir Immune Defic Syndr* 1991; 4:659-66.

[64] Yajko DM, Nassos PS, Hadley WK. Therapeutic implications of inhibition versus killing of Mycobacterium avium complex by antimicrobial agents. *Antimicrob Agents Chemother* 1987; 31:117-20.

[65] Yajko DM, Kirihara J, Sanders C, Nassos P, Hadley WK. Antimicrobial synergism against *Mycobacterium avium* complex strains isolated from patients with acquired immune deficiency syndrome. *Antimicrob Agents Chemother* 1988; 32:1392-5.

[66] Fernandes PB, Hardy DJ, McDaniel D, Hanson CW, Swanson RN. *In vitro* and *in vivo* activities of clarithromycin against *Mycobacterium avium. Antimicrob Agents Chemother* 1989; 33:1531-4.

[67] Inderlied CB, Kolonoski PT, Wu M, Young LS. Amikacin, ciprofloxacin, and imipenem treatment for disseminated *Mycobacterium avium* complex infection of beige mice. *Antimicrob Agents Chemother* 1989; 33:176-80.

[68] Cohn DL, Fisher EJ, Peng GT, et al. A prospective randomized trial of four three-drug regimens in the treatment of disseminated *Mycobacterium avium* complex disease in AIDS patients: excess mortality associated with high-dose clarithromycin. *Clin Infect Dis* 1999; 29:125-33.

[69] Kemper CA, Havlir D, Haghighat D, et al. The individual microbiologic effect of three antimycobacterial agents, clofazimine, ethambutol, and rifampin, on *Mycobacterium avium* complex bacteremia in patients with AIDS. *J Infect Dis* 1994; 170:157-64.

[70] Chaisson RE, Keiser P, Pierce M, et al. Clarithromycin and ethambutol with or without clofazimine for the treatment of bacteremic *Mycobacterium avium* complex disease in patients with HIV infection. *AIDS* 1997; 11:311-7.

[71] Parenti DM, Williams PL, Hafner R, et al. A phase II/III trial of antimicrobial therapy with or without amikacin in the treatment of disseminated *Mycobacterium avium* infection in HIV-infected individuals. *AIDS* 1998; 12:2439-46.

[72] El-Sadr WM, Burman WJ, Grant LB, et al. Discontinuation of prophylaxis for *Mycobacterium avium* complex disease in HIV-infected patients who have a response to antiretroviral therapy. *N Engl J Med 2000*; 342:1085-92.

[73] Currier JS, Williams PL, Koletar SL, et al. Discontinuation of *Mycobacterium avium* complex prophylaxis in patients with antiretroviral therapy-induced increases in CD4+ cell count. A randomized, double-blind, placebo-controlled trial. AIDS Clinical Trials Group 362 Study Team. *Ann Intern Med* 2000; 133:493-503.

[74] Shelburne SA, Visnegarwala F, Darcourt J, et al. Incidence and risk factors for immune reconstitution inflammatory syndrome during highly active antiretroviral therapy. *AIDS* 2005; 19:399-406.

[75] Lipman M, Breen R. Immune reconstitution inflammatory syndrome in HIV. *Curr*

Opin Infect Dis 2006; 19:20-5.

[76] Hirsch HH, Kaufmann G, Sendi P, Battegay M. Immune reconstitution in HIV-infected patients. *Clin Infect Dis* 2004; 38:1159-66.

[77] Tuon FF, Mulatti GC, Pinto WP, De Siqueira Franca FO, Grysheck RC. Immune reconstitution inflammatory syndrome associated with disseminated mycobacterial infection in patients with AIDS. *AIDS Patient Care STDs* 2007; 21:527-32.

In: AIDS- Related Opportunistic Infections
Editor: Claudia D. Galanda
ISBN: 978-1-60692-144-9

Chapter III

HIV Infection and Pneumocystis Pneumonia (PCP)

Jose G. Castro and Luis Espinoza
University of Miami, Coral Gables, Florida, USA

Abstract

Pneumocystis pneumonia (PCP) or pneumocystosis remains as one of the most prevalent opportunistic infections in patients infected with the human immunodeficiency virus (HIV) and remains as one of the most common causes death in patients with AIDS. Pneumocystosis in humans is caused by to *P. jiroveci*, different from *P. carinii* that is one of the two *Pneumocystis* species found only in rats. First was identified as a protozoan nearly 100 years ago, it has been reclassified as a fungus, in 1988, based on DNA analysis. *P. jiroveci* has worldwide distribution among humans and has been detected in a variety of animals. It is difficult to find in the environment and has not been found in nonhuman hosts. It is absent or present a very low levels in healthy adults, in contrast, it is fairly common in immunocompromised individuals. *Pneumocystis* is acquired by airborne route and takes up residence in the alveoli adhering to type I cells. In immunocompromised hosts it propagates and fills the alveoli. It results in increased alveolar-capillary permeability and damage to type I cells. There is alteration on the pulmonary surfactant and, in severe disease, may include interstitial edema, fibrosis, and hyaline membrane formation. The clinical picture is quite variable. Most patients are usually ill for two to three weeks. Progressive dyspnea is characteristic, but dry cough, tachycardia, tachypnea, cyanosis, and low-grade fever are also common manifestations. Lung auscultation is usually unremarkable. Arterial blood gas demonstrates hypoxia, increased alveolar-arterial gradient and respiratory alkalosis. Desaturation on exercise of $\geq$ 5% is a reliable and quick test. Chest radiography classically shows fine, bilateral, diffuse infiltrates beginning in the perihilar regions. Early in the disease the chest radiography may be normal. Other presentations include unilateral infiltrates, cavitary lesions, nodular densities, cystic formation, pleural effusion, pneumothorax, and pneumomediastinum. High resolution computerized tomography is more sensitive than chest radiography in the diagnosis of PCP. Definitive diagnosis is based on specific identification of the organism by histopathologic staining. Sputum induction has wide variety of success. In seven prospective studies demonstrated 55.5% sensitivity and 98.6% specificity. Fiber optic bronchoscopy with bronchoalveolar lavage has > 90% sensitivity and 100% specificity. The drug of choice is trimethoprim-sulfamethoxazole (TMP-SMZ) and in severe cases it is recommended the concomitant use of steroids. Alternative drugs include: Atovaquone, clindamycin, primaquine, dapsone plus trimethoprim and pentamidine

1. Introduction

Pneumocystis jiroveci, previously known as *Pneumocystis carinii*, is the organism responsible for *Pneumocystis carinii* pneumonia (PCP); the most common opportunistic infection (OI) in HIV-infected patients. Before the advent of the acquired immunodeficiency syndrome (AIDS) epidemic, in the early 1980s, *Pneumocystis carinii* pneumonia was a rare infection (less than 100 cases per year in the US) seem mainly in immunosuppressed patients with protein malnutrition or malignancies, [1,2] or in patients receiving corticosteroid therapy. [3] For example, an epidemic of interstitial plasma cell pneumonia was reported in premature and malnourished children, particularly those in orphanages in Europe in the late 1930's and early 1940's. [4] Another epidemic of *P. carinii* pneumonia was described in the 1960's in children with congenital defects of the immune system and in children and adults with acquired defects of the immune system secondary to malignancy or its treatment. Later, the relationship of *P. carinii* pneumonia with immunosuppression became evident in organ transplant patients. In 1981, the Centers for Disease Control and Prevention (CDC) reported the occurrence of PCP in 5 previously healthy homosexual males residing in the Los Angeles area. This outbreak will become one of the initial signs of the emergence of AIDS pandemic[4] . Few years later, PCP became both the most frequent index diagnosis in patients with HIV infection and the most common OI in HIV-infected patients: PCP was diagnosed in up to 75% of patients with AIDS. [5,6] This sudden increase of cases with high mortality rate in previously healthy individuals stimulated both basic and clinical research. Few years later, important advances were accomplished in the understanding, management and prevention of this otherwise fatal infection. For example, the use of prophylaxis for the prevention of PCP became the standard of care in the management of HIV infection in 1987, as well as the concomitant use of steroids and antibiotics in the management of severe PCP cases. In the last few years, the incidence and fatality rate of PCP has decreased: earlier diagnosis of HIV infection, widespread use of potent antiretroviral therapy and effective prophylaxis have all contributed to a 75 percent decline in cases, although PCP remains the most common AIDS-defining illness.

2. Etiology

The full identification and classification of Pneumocystis took many decades. The organism was first described in 1909 by Chagas, with the use of a guinea-pig model of trypanosome infection and subsequently by Antonio Carinii, in the infected rat lungs. [7,8] Few years later Delanöes [9] isolated the organism from rats and realized that this organism was a new specie and ultimately named the organism *Pneumocystis carinii* given its unique tropism for the lung and also in the honor of Dr Carini. Years later, Dr Otto Jirovec and his group isolated the organism from humans, and it is after him that the organism responsible for PCP pneumonia was recently renamed. Pneumocystis is an eukaryotic microorganism that is found worldwide. The genus *Pneumocystis* is composed of multiple individual species that require an specific mammalian host. Its host range is wide and include humans and other mammals such as rabbits, [10] dogs, [11] goats, [12] swine, [13] cats, [14] chimpanzees, [15] owl monkeys, [16] and horses. [17] The specific species that infect humans is named *Pneumocystis jirovecii* (previously known as *Pneumocystis carinii f. sp. Hominis*). [18] Distinct genomic variability exists between host-specific members of the genus.

Microbiology

The taxonomic classification of the *Pneumocystis* genus was debated for some time. It was initially mistaken as a trypanosome and later as a protozoan. It was believed to be a protozoan because of its three morphologic forms: cysts, sporozoites and trophozoites. Cysts are round or crescent shaped, five to eight microns in diameter, and covered by a three-layer pellicle. The mature cysts can contain up to eight sporozoites, which are crescent-shaped intracystic structures one to two microns in diameter. Trophozoites are the free-floating forms of Pneumocystis. These trophozoites are two to five microns in size and are pleomorphic. They tend to form clusters and resemble platelets. In the 1980s, biochemical analysis of the nucleic acid composition of *Pneumocystis* rRNA disclosed homology to the one found in fungi rather than the one in protozoa. [19,20] Additionally, ultrastructural studies of Pneumocystis failed to demonstrate the cytoskeletal elements and complex organelle systems, peculiar of protozoa. [21] Subsequent genomic sequence analysis of multiple genes including elongation factor 3, a component of fungi protein synthesis not found in protozoa, further supported the hyphotesis that *Pneumocystis* is a fungus.

3. Pathogenesis

Serological studies have demonstrated that *P.jirovecci* infection occurs relatively early in life. [22,23] This idea has been confirmed with longitudinal studies that have demosntrated the presence of this infection early in life, with seroconversion demonstrated in 85% of children by 20 months of age. [24] A better understanding of the natural history of *P jiroveci* infection has come from recent animal studies showing a typical pattern of infection, transmission and resolution in immunologically normal hosts. [25] It is also becoming more apparent that PCP results from a new infection rather than reactivation of a latent infection, since no latency has ever been demonstrated, and mouse and rat models of PCP have shown that latency does not develop after infection. [26,27] The actual mode of transmission is unknown, but it is probably limited to aerosol route, [28] with cysts expelled during exhalation and coughing. Cysts are then inhalated by another individual. In the pulmonary alveoli, intracystic bodies are released and developed into trophozoites. These trophozoites attach and interdigitate with type I [29,30] and possibly type II pneumocytes. [31,32] The alveolar surface lining layer, composed of phospholipids, apoproteins, mucopolysaccharides and surfactant, may nourish and even protect the organism. It is believed that attachment to the alveolar epithelium is required for Pneumocystis proliferation, because studies in which attachment was prevented by physical or chemical means, proliferation was inhibited. [33] An effective host inflammatory response is required to eliminate Pneumocystis infection. However the normal host has to produce a perfectly balanced immune response, since a vigorous inflammatory response to Pneumocystis will produce exuberant inflammation that will promote pulmonary injury. Indeed, PCP is characterized by lung inflammation involving neutrophils and $CD8^+$ T cells, which induce diffuse alveolar damage and impair gas exchange, leading to respiratory failure. For example, respiratory impairment and death are more closely correlated to the extend of lung inflammation than to the severity of the organism burden present during PCP. [34]

Host response is then, a major determinant of disease severity. As described above, prior to the advent of AIDS epidemic, most cases of PCP occurred in patients receiving treatment for malignancies. The initial observations underscoring the importance of the degree of immune response as the main factor determining the clinical manifestations of PCP were: occurrence of PCP after the cessation of corticosteroid therapy and, in bone marrow transplant patients, emergence of PCP typically followed by evidence of engraftment. These two observations raised the question of whether the manifestation of PCP was enhanced as the immunosuppressed host acquired some ability to mount an immune response. With numerous cases available during the AIDS epidemic, it became clear that the clinical manifestations of PCP were different between AIDS and non AIDS patients. PCP occurs in AIDS patients when they develop advance immunosuppression manifested by a marked loss of CD4+ T cells. Patients with AIDS develop PCP with a more subtle, insidious presentation; have lower respiratory rates and higher arterial oxygen tensions than patients with other immunosuppressive conditions, largely hematological conditions. [35] Additionally, the mortality rate for PCP in AIDS patients is 5-10%, compared to about 40% in non-AIDS patients. [36] This lower PCP-associated mortality in AIDS patients occurs despite the fact that these patients typically have higher organism burdens than patients with malignancies. [37]

Macrophage activity: Alveolar macrophages are the primary resident phagocytes that mediate the clearance of microorganisms from the lung. The uptake of Pneumocystis by macrophages occurs through multiple receptor systems. The normal macrophage function is impaired in patients with AIDS and in patients with malignancies, resulting in suppressed clearance of Pneumocystis infection. [38] In addition to degrading Pneumocystis, alveolar macrophages also produce a large variety of pro-inflammatory chemokines, cytokines and additional inflammatory mediators following interaction with Pneumocystis. [38] These mediators generally participate in eradicating Pneumocystis but also promote lung injury.

Lymphocyte responses during PCP: The host immune response during PCP involves complex interactions between $CD4^+$ T cells, CD8 $^+$ T cells, neutrophils, alveolar macrophages and soluble mediators that facilitate clearance of the infection. However, the central role in the host defense against Pneumocystis is played by the $CD4^+$ T cells, both in humans and in animal models of infection, and highlighted by the increased risk of infection in patients with $CD4^+$ T-cell counts bellow 200 per μL. [39,40] $CD4^+$T cells provide essential memory-cell functions that coordinate the host inflammatory response by recruiting and activating additional immune effector cells including monocytes and macrophages, which are responsible for elimination of the organism. It has been shown [41] that macrophage-derived TNF and IL-1, which are released following direct interaction with the organism, are required for the initiation of the $CD4^+$ T cells response during PCP, furthermore, $CD4^+$T cells proliferate in response to Pneumocystis antigens and generate cytokines, including IFN- γ and lymphotactin.

Cytokines: several cytokines and chemokines are involved in the control of Pneumocystis infection but the three better studied are: IL-8, TNF-α and IFN γ. For example, IL-8 production is correlated with neutrophil infiltration of the lung and impaired gas exchange during severe PCP. The level of IL-8 detected in bronchoalveolar lavage fluid could predict the severity of respiratory compromise and death from PCP in humans. [42] These cytokines are released when various components on the Pneumocystis cell surface stimulate lung cells, including macrophages and epithelial cells. One of these components is a β-glucan molecule. Accumulating evidence indicates that innate recognition of this cell-wall component is an important early factor driving the initiation of lung inflammation during PCP. [43,44]

4. Epidemiology

There has been a dramatic change in the epidemiology of Pneumocystis pneumonia in the last 30 years: With the advent of the HIV/AIDS epidemic in the early 1980's there was a sudden increase in cases of PCP; later followed by a significant decrease, probably related to the widespread use of PCP prophylaxis first, and later (1996) to the availability of potent antiretroviral therapy. [45] In the other hand, given the increased number of patients undergoing transplants and receiving chemotherapy, it has been a gradual increase of cases of PCP in non-HIV infected individuals. For example, there was a report of increased incidence of PCP requiring intensive care unit admission in HIV-negative patients from 1993 to 2006 in a Hospital in France. [46]

The prevalence of PCP was once thought to be much lower in developing regions of the world, but newer studies have shown that the lower incidence reported is likely a failure of accurately diagnose the condition rather than paucity of cases. Accurate diagnosis, as described in the next section, requires access to modern medical care not always available worldwide. For example a report from Africa describes up to 80% of HIV-infected infants with Pneumocystis.

5. Clinical Manifestations

The clinical presentation of PCP seems to be different in HIV infected compared to non-HIV infected patients. Patients who have pneumocystis pneumonia without AIDS typically present with an abrupt onset of respiratory insufficiency that may correlate with a tapered or increased dose of immunosupressant medications. [47,48] The mortality rate among these patients is 30 to 60 percent, depending on the population at risk, with a greater risk of death among patients with cancer than among patients undergoing transplantation or those with connective-tissue disease. [49,50] In HIV infected individuals, patients usually have minimal symptoms and a normal physical exam at rest when seen early in the course of their PCP. As the pneumonia progresses, generally patients report a gradual onset of symptoms (Several days to two week) characterized by fever, cough, and progressive dyspnea. [51] The cough is generally nonproductive, but as many as 30 percent of patients may have some sputum production. On the other hand, patients may present with more advanced disease or even when they are on the brink of respiratory failure. Another presentation of which clinicians should be aware is pneumothorax. Finding pneumothorax in an HIV-infected patient with no other precipitating cause should raise the possibility of PCP, especially if the patient is receiving aerosolized pentamidine. [52,53] Overall, the most common findings on physical examination are fever, tachycardia and tachypnea. A normal chest exam occurs in 50 percent of the cases. Pneumocystis infection is not only confined to the lungs, but may also be disseminated via lymphatics and hematogenous routes. [54,55] These extrapulmonary manifestations are uncommon., but typically involves thyroid, liver, bone marrow, lymph nodes, and spleen. [55,56] These manifestations seem to be more common in patients receiving aerosolized pentamidine as PCP prophylaxis.

6. Diagnosis

Pneumocystis pneumonia may be difficult to diagnose owing to nospecific symptoms and signs, the use of prophylactic drugs in the treatment of HIV-infected patients, simultaneous infections with multiple organisms (such as cytomegalovirus, [57] mycobacterium tuberculosis [58]) and the widespread practice of empiric treatment of PCP in patients with HIV infection presenting with pneumonia. [59,60] Typical radiographic features of PCP are bilateral interstitial infiltrates that become increasingly homogeneous and diffuse as the disease progresses (Fig 1,2,3). However, almost every conceivable radiographic pattern has been reported with PCP, including lobar infiltrates, cavities, upper lobe predominance, asymmetrical patterns, pneumothorax and up to 25% of normal chest radiograph at presentation. Upper lobe infiltrates are reportedly more common in patients receiving aerosolized pentamidine. When chest radiograph are normal, high resolution computed tomography may reveal extensive ground-glass attenuation or cystic lesions. [61] Gallium-67 citrate scanning is a highly sensitive test in patients with PCP, demonstrating intense, diffuse bilateral uptake, [62] however its role is limited by lack of specificity, its high cost, and a two-day delay in obtaining final results. Nevertheless, it may have some usefulness as a screening test when there is a question of active pulmonary infection, especially in patients with normal pulmonary radiographs. The assessment of oxygenation at rest and with exercise is, however, a valuable screening test. [63] The presence of PCP is highly unlikely if the response to exercise is normal. The two most common abnormal laboratory values associated with PCP in patients with HIV infection are a CD4 count bellow 200 cells/mm^3 and an elevated lactate deshydrogenase (LDH) level. [64-66] The elevation of LDH it is likely a reflection of the underlying lung inflammation and injury rather than a specific marker for the disease. [67] However, establishing a definitive diagnosis of the cause of penumonia is recommended. For example, in the era of widespread use of antiretrovirals, PCP is less common and may have atypical presentations, and therapy may be toxic or contraindicated (For example the use of steroids in patients with presumed to have PCP but actually infected with Mycobacterium tuberculosis [58]). The definitive diagnosis of PCP requires documentation of the organism from a clinically relevant source, because pneumocystis can not be cultivated.

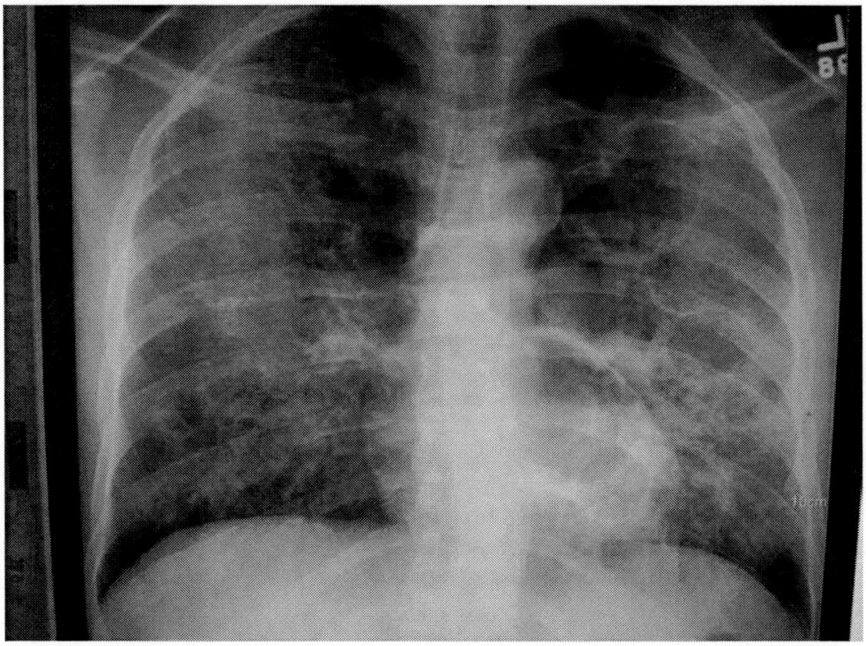

Figure 1. Chest radiograph of a patient with PCP showing bilateral infiltrates and multiple bullas.

A. Sputum induction. Sputum induction with hypertonic saline has a diagnostic yield of 50 to 90 percent and a specificity approaching 100 percent. [68,69] It should be the initial procedure used to diagnose pneumocystis pneumonia, particularly in patients with AIDS. A study [70] reported an increase of the sensitivity of this test up to 95% with the use of immunofluorecent staining. This technique uses monoclonal antibodies against glycoproteins in the cell walls of the cysts and trophozoites of pneumocystis to increase the diagnostic yield of the test.

B. *Bronchoscopy*. If the initial specimen of induced sputum is negative for pneumocystis or can not be performed (patient can not cooperate, is too dyspneic, has altered mental status) then bronchoscopy with bronchoalveolar lavage should be performed. Transbronschoscopic or surgical lung biopsy is rarely needed. [71]. Trophic forms can be detected with modified Papanicolau, Wright-Giemsa, or Gram-Weigert stains. Cuts can be stained with Gomori methenamine silver, cresyl echt violet, toluidine blue O, or calcofluor white. The use of monoclonal antibodies does not increase much the sensitivity of these stains, [72] but provides the advantage of staining both, trophic forms and cysts, which is important because the trophic forms are generally more abundant during pneumocystis pneumonia.

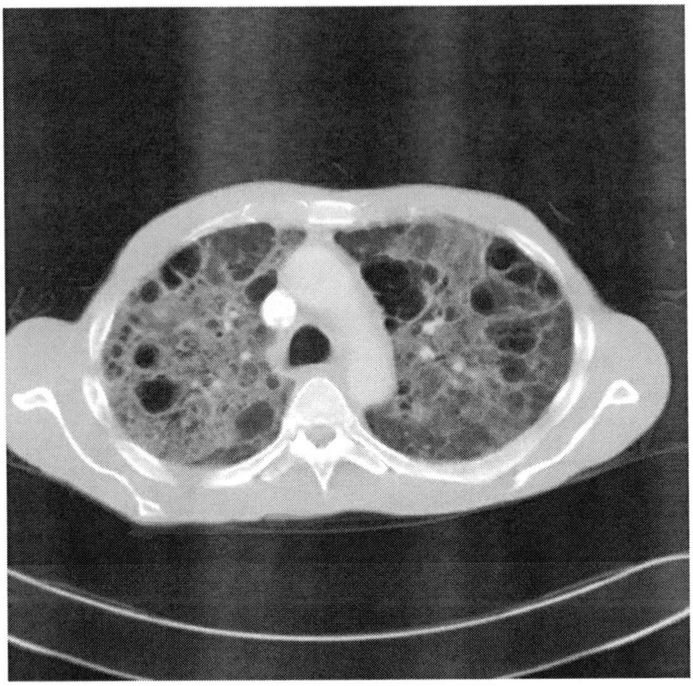

Figure 2. Chest Computed tomography of a patient with PCP showing multiple cysts and bilateral interstitial infiltrates.

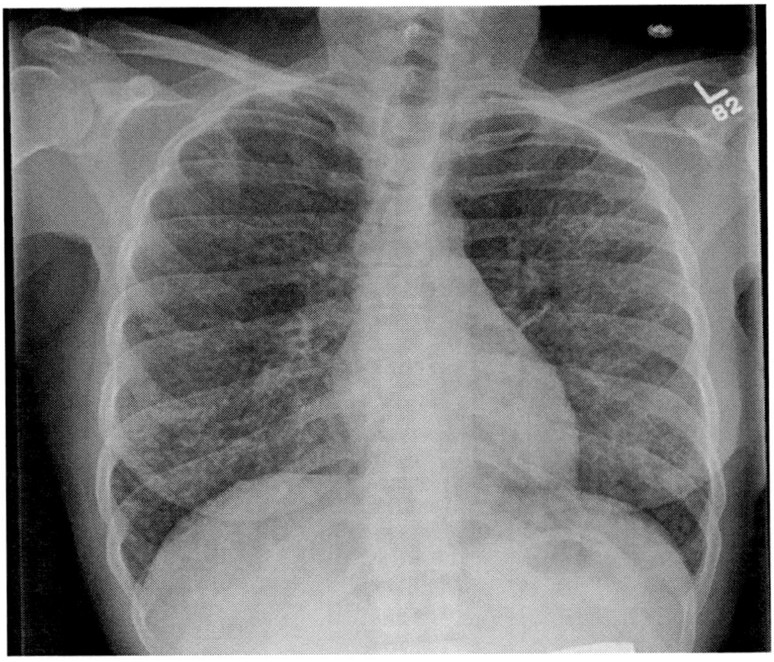

Figure 3. Typical Chest radiograph of a patient with PCP with bilateral interstitial infiltrates

C. *Newer tests*. The use of polymerase chain reaction (PCR) to detect pneumocystis nucleic acids has been an area of active research. PCR has been shown to have greater sensitivity and specificity for the diagnosis of pneumocystis pneumonia from specimens of induced sputum and bronchoalveolar lavage than conventional staining methods. [73,74] Additionally, this method could allow quantification of the organism in the attempt to differentiate colonization from infection and could be used to detect drug resistance. [75,76] A recent pilot study, [77] reported lower levels of S-adenosylmethionine in blood in patients with confirmed pneumocystis pneumonia compared to normal levels detected in patients with other pulmonary infections. Additionally, the concentrations rose within one week in patients who responded to therapy. Further studies will be needed to confirm these preliminary findings.

7. Treatment

The drug of choice for pneumocystosis is trimethoprim-sulfamethoxazole (TMP-SMX) which is available in oral and parenteral forms. These drugs target the dihydrofolate reductase and dihydropteroate synthase respectively. Therapeutic failure occurs in up to 20% of the cases, mostly related to adverse events. Actually, adverse reactions to this combination have been observed in more than one half of the cases and treatment limiting toxicities in one third of the cases. [78] Reported toxicities include skin reaction (ranging from mild rash to anaphylaxis), drug fever, nephritis, bone marrow suppression, nausea and vomiting, diarrhea, pancreatitis, metabolic acidosis, and hyperkalemia.

Resistance to TMP-SMX is considerate rare and if occurs it is caused by mutations in the dihydropteroate synthase. The recommended dose for the treatment of PCP is 15 to 20 mg/kg of TMP per day and 75 to 100 mg/kg of SMX per day divided in three or four doses. The length of treatment is 21 days in HIV-infected patients and 14 days in non-HIV infected individuals. However the duration of the recommended therapy may be longer if there is a delay in the resolution of signs and symptoms. [79] The reason for longer duration of treatment in HIV infected individuals is due to the larger burden of organisms and the slower response to the therapy. The dose of these medications needs to be adjusted in case of renal or hepatic impairment.

In patients who have allergy or intolerance to sulfonamides, there are several alternatives including dapsone 100 mg orally daily plus trimethoprim 15 mg/kg daily orally divided in 3 doses. Its efficacy is similar to TMP/SMX with less toxicity. Adverse reactions include hemolysis in patients who have glucose 6 phosphate dehydrogenase (G6PD) deficiency, methemoglobinemia, rash, fever, nausea and vomiting.

Another comparable alternative to the above regimens include the use of clindamycin 300-450 mg orally four times a day (600-900 mg IV every 6 to 8 hours) plus primaquine 15-30 mg of base daily. The mechanism of action of both drugs against Pneumocystis is unknown. The most common adverse reactions include skin rash, gastrointestinal complaints, and fever. Primaquine may also cause hemolysis in patients with G6PD deficiency.

Atovaquone, an antimalarial agent, has also activity against *Pneumocystis* although is less effective than the above regimens. Its efficacy is similar to the one of pentamidine. The usual dose is in suspension, 750 mg orally twice daily, taken with food to increase its absorption. Adverse reactions include skin rash, fever, gastrointestinal symptoms, and abnormal liver function tests. Muations in the cytochrome b gene have been shown to confer resistance to atovaquone. [80]

Pentamidine isethionate was first used to treat African trypanosomiasis, and its precise mechanism of action against *Pneumocystis* is unknown. Pentamidine is usually given via intravenous route at 4 mg/kg once daily. The aerosol route is recommended for prophylaxis but not treatment of PCP. It is a highly toxic drug and major side effects include hypotension, cardiac arrhythmias, electrolytes abnormalities, hypo and hyperglycemias, bronchospasm, etc.

Trimetrexate is a folate antagonist with activity against *Pneumocystis*, and the recommended dose is 45 mg/m2 once daily intravenous. It must be administered with concurrent leucovorin to avoid serious life-threatening toxicities and it must be extended for 72 hours past the last dose of trimetrexate. The leucovorin dose is 20 mg/m2 every 6 hours. However trimetrexate is not longer available in the US since its production has been discontinued in March 2007.

In cases of severe PCP (defined as an arterial oxygen pressure of less than 70 mmHg or an alveolar-arterial gradient greater than 35 mmHg) it is recommended the concomitant use of steroids. These steroids should be use ideally prior to the first dose of antibiotics or not later than the first 72 hours of the initiation of therapy. The usual dose of steroids is prednisone 40 mg orally twice daily for the first five days, 40 mg orally daily for another five days, 20 mg orally for the following 11 days. If intravenous therapy is necessary then methylprednisolone at 75% of respective prednisolone should be administered. The reason for this recommendation is because it have been shown that the use of steroids in addition to the specific therapy improves the outcome specially because frequently there is a deterioration in the oxygenation during the first days of therapy, probably due to an inflammatory response from the dying organisms. [81]

Patients with severe PCP frequently develop respiratory failure and require mechanical ventilation and admission to intensive care units. With improvements in the management of these patients, there has been a gradual improvement in survival in these cases in the last two decades. [82-84]

8. Prevention

Primary Prophylaxis

It is indicated for persons with HIV infection and a CD4 count of less than 200 cells/mm^3 (or CD4/CD8 ratio of less than 14%) or those with recurrent oropharyngeal candidiasis. Patients at risk for PCP, who are not infected by HIV, include those with hematologic malignancics, solid tumors, inflammatory disorders, and post-bone marrow or solid organ transplantation. [85] For these groups of patients there is not an established recommended regimen but it is accepted to be the same than in advanced HIV infection. Patients who

develop PCP while on prophylaxis have a poor outcome from severe PCP may be due to acquired co-trimoxazole resistance. [86,87]
The following are the recommended regimens:

- TMP-SMZ one Double Strength tablet orally daily or three times a week, or one single-strength tablet orally daily (preferred).
- Dapsone 100 mg orally daily
- Dapsone 50 mg orally daily with pyrimethamine 50 mg orally weekly plus folinic acid 25 mg orally weekly
- Atovaquone suspension 750 mg orally twice daily
- Aerosolized pentamidine 300 mg every four weeks administered via Respirgard II® nebulizer

Primary prophylaxis may be discontinued in patients on antiretroviral therapy whose CD4 counts are above 200 cells/mm^3 for at least three months. It should be re-introduced if CD4 count decreases to less than 200 cells/mm^3

Secondary Prophylaxis

Patients with a history of PCP should have chemoprophylaxis with any of the above mentioned regimens for life unless immune reconstitution occurs. If the CD4 count rises above 200 cells/mm^3 for at least three months in response to HAART, then it may be discontinued. Secondary prophylaxis should be restarted if the CD4 count declines to less than 200 cells/mm^3 or if PCP recurred with CD4 counts above 200 cells/mm^3.[79]

9. Conclusion

PCP remains as one of the most common and most deadly opportunistic infections in patients with Human Immunodeficiency Virus infection. It is also becoming more common in non-HIV infected individuals as the number of patients undergoing chemotherapy and immunosuppresion after transplant is growing. Clinicians need to become familiar with its presentation and management because mild cases can be difficult to diagnose but severe cases may need care in intensive care units with mechanical ventilation and can even be fatal. Currently, the most effective medication for its prevention and treatment is trimethoprim-sulfamethoxazole but few other alternative medications are alsoavailable.

10. References

[1] Rosen P, Armstrong D, Ramos C. *Pneumocystis carinii* pneumonia: a clinicopathologic study of twenty patients with neoplastic diseases. Am J Med. 1972;53:428-436.

[2] Hughes WT, Price RA, Kim HK, et al. *Pneumocystis carinii* pneumonitis in children with malignancies. J Pediatr. 1973;82:404-415.

[3] Yale SH, Limper AH. *Pneumocystis carinii* pneumonia in patients without acquired immunodeficiency syndrome: associated illnesses and prior corticosteroid therapy. Mayo Clin Proc. 1996; 71:5-13.

[4] Hughes WT, Prologue to AIDS: the recognition of infectious opportunists. Medicine (Baltimore). 198;77:227-232.

[5] Hoover DR, Saah AJ, Bacellar H, et al. Clinical manifestations of AIDS in the era of *Pneumocystis* prophylaxis. Multicenter AIDS Cohort Study. *N Engl J Med.* 1993; 329:1922-1926.

[6] Levine SJ. *Pneumocystis carinii. Clin Chest Med.* 1996;17:665-695.

[7] Chagas C. Nova tripanozomiaze humana: estudo sobre a morfolojia e o evolutivo do Schizotrypanum cruzi n.gen.,sp., ajente etiolojico de nova entidade morbida do homem. Mem Inst Oswaldo Cruz 1909;1:159-218.

[8] Carinii A. Formas de eschizogonia do Trypanozoma lewisi. Commun Soc Med Sao Paolo 1910;16:204.

[9] Delanoe P, Delanoe M. Sur les rapports des kystes de Carini du poumon des rats avec le Trypanosoma Lewisi. C R Acad Sci 1912;155:658-60.

[10] Sheldon WH. Experimental pulmonary Pneumocystis carinii in rabbits. J Exp Med. 1959;110:147-160.

[11] Copland JW. Canine pneumonia caused by Pneumocustis carinii. Aust Vet J. 1974;50:515-518.

[12] McConnell EE, Basson PA, Pienaar JG. Pneumocystis in domestic goat. Ondertepoort J Vet Res. 1971;38:117-124.

[13] Siebold HR, Munnell JF. Pneumocystis in pig. Vet Pathol. 1977;14:89..

[14] Settness OP, Hasselager E. Occurrence of Pneumocystis carinii. Delanoe & Delanoe, 1912 in dogs and cats in Denmark. Nord Vet Med. 1984;36:179-181.

[15] Chandler FW, McClure HM, Campbell WG, Watss JC. Pulmonary pneumocustosis in nonhuman primates. Arch Pathol Lab Med. 1976;100:163-167.

[16] Long GG, White JD, Stookey JL. Pneumocystis carinii infection in splenectomized owl monkeys. J Am Vet Med Assoc. 1975;167:651-654.

[17] Shively JN, Moe KK, Dellers RW. Fine structure of spontaneous Pneumocystis carinii pulmonary infection in foals. Cornell Vet. 1974;64:72-88.

[18] Stringer JR, Beard CB, Miller RF, Wakefield AE. A new name (Pneumocystis jiroveci) for Pneumocystis from humans. Emerg Infect Dis. 2002;8:891-896.

[19] Edman JC, Kovacs JA, Masur H, Santi DV, et al. Ribosomal RNA sequence shows Pneumocystis carinii to be a member of fungi. Natue. 1988;334:519-522.

[20] Stringer SL, Hudson K, Blasé MA, Walzer PD, et al. Sequence from ribosomal RNA of Pneumocystis carinii compared to those of four fungi suggests an ascomycettous affinity. J Protozool. 1989;36:14S-16S.

[21] Bedrossian CWM. Rapid cytologic diagnosis of Penumocystis: a comparison of effective techniques. Semin Diagn Pathol. 1989;6(3)245-261.

[22] Peglow SL, et al. Serologic responses to Pneumocystis carinii antigens in health and disease. J Infect Dis. 1990;161:296-306.

[23] Meuwissen JH. Infections with Pneumocystis carinii. Natl Cancer Inst Monogr. 1976;43:133-6.

[24] Vargas SL, et al. Search for primary infection by Pneumocystis carinii in a cohort of normal, healthy infants. Clin Infect Dis. 2001;32:855-861.

[25] Gigliotti F, Harmsen AG, and Wright TW. Characterization of transmission of Pneumocystis carinii f. sp. Muris through immunocompetent BALB/c mice. Infect Immun 2003;71:3852-56.

[26] Chen W, Gigliotti F, and Harmsen AG. Latency is not an inevitable outcome of infection with Pneumocystis carinii. Infect Immun. 1993;61:5406-9.

[27] Vargas SL, et al. Limited persistence in and subsequent elimination of *Pneumocystis carinii* from the lungs after *P. carinii* pneumonia. 1995;172:506-10.

[28] Hughes WT, Bartley DL, and Smith BM. A natural source of infection of Pneumocystis carinii. J Infect Dis 1983;117:595.

[29] Henshaw NG, Carson JL and Collier AM. Ultrastructural observations of Pneumocystis carinii attachment to the lung. J Infect Dis 1985;151:181-6.

[30] Itatani CA, Marshall GJ. Ultrastructural morphology and staining characteristics of Pneumocystis carinii in situ and from bronchioalveolar lavage J Parasitol 1988;74:700-12.

[31] Long EG, Smith JS, and Meier JL. Attachment of Pneumocystis carinii to rat pneumocytes. Lab Invest 1986;54:609-15.

[32] Millard PR, Wakefield AE, and Hopkins JM. A sequential ultrastructural study of rat lungs infected with Pneumocystis carinii to investigate the appareance of the organism, its relationships and its effects on pneumocytes. Int J Exp Pathol 1990;71:895-904.

[33] Limper AH, Martin WJ. Pneumocystis carinii: inhibition of lung cell growth mediated by parasite attachment. J Clin Invest 1990;85:391-6.

[34] Limper AH, Offord KP, Smith TF and WJ 2nd. Pneumocystis carinii pneumonia. Differences in lung parasite number and inflammation in patients with and without AIDS. Am Rev Respir Dis 1989;140:1204-9.

[35] Kovacs JA, et al. Pneumocystis carinii pneumonia: a comparison between patients with the acquired immunodeficiency syndrome and patients with other immunodeficiencies. Ann Intern Med 1984;100:663-671.

[36] Mansharamani NG, et al. Management and outcome patterns for adult Pneumocystis carinii pneumonia, 1985 to 1995: comparison of HIV associated cases to other immunocompromised states. Chest 2000;118:704-711.

[37] Ziefer A and Abramowitz JA. Pneumocystis carinii pneumonia in HIV-positive and HIV-negative patients. An epidemiological, clinical and histopathological study of 18 patients. S Afr med J 1989;76:308-313.

[38] Limper AH, Hoyte JS and Standing JE. The role of alveolar macrophages in Pneumocystis carinii degradation and clearance from the lung. J Clin Invest 1997;99:2110-7.

[39] Phair J, et al. The risk of Pneumocystis carinii pneumonia among men infected with human immunodeficiency virus type 1. Multicenter AIDS Cohort Study Group. N. Eng J Med 1990;322:161-5.

[40] Shellito J, et al. A new model of Pneumocystis carinii infection in mice selectively depleted of helper T lymphocytes. L Clin Invest 1990;85:1686-93.

[41] Beck JM and Harmsen AG. Lymphocytes in host defense against Pneumocystis carinii. Semin Respir 1998;13:330-8.

[42] Benfield TL, et al. Prognostic value of interleukin-8 in AIDS associated Pneumocystis carinii pneumonia. Am J respire Crit Care Med. 995;151:1058-62.

[43] Carmona EM, et al. Pneumocystis cell wall β-glucans induce dendritic cell costimulatory molecule expression and inflammatory activation through a Fas-fas ligand mechanism. J Immunol 2006;177:459-67.

[44] Hahn PY et al. Pneumocystis carinii cell wall β-glucan induces release of macrophage inflammatory protein-2 from alveolar epithelial cells via a lactosylceramide-mediated mechanism J Biol Chem 2003;278:2043-50.

[45] Kaplan JE, Hanson D, Dworkin MS, et al. Epidemiology of human immunodeficiency virus-associated opportunistic infections in the United States in the era of highly active antiretroviral therapy. CID 2000; 30:S5-14.

[46] Monnet X, Vidal-Petiot E, Osman D, et al. Critical care management and outcome of severe Pneumocystis pneumonia in patients with and without HIV infection. Critical Care 2008, 12:R28 (25 January 2008).

[47] Sepkowitz KA, Brown AE, Telzak EE, Gottlieb S, Armstrong D. Pneumocystis carinii pneumonia among patients without AIDS at a cancer hospital. JAMA 1992;267:832-7.

[48] Yale SH, Limper AH. Pneumocystis carinii pneumonia in patients without acquired immunodeficiency síndrome:associated illness and prior corticosteroid therapy. Mayo Clin Proc 1996;71:5-13.

[49] Sepkowitz KA. Opportunistic infections in patients with and patients without acquired immunodeficiency síndrome. Clin Infect Dise 2002;34:1098-107.

[50] Pareja JG, Garland R, Koziel H. Use of adjuntive corticosteroids in severe adult non-HIV Pneumocystis carinii pneumonia. Chest 1998;113:1215-24.

[51] Kales CP, Murren JR, Torres RA, Crocco JA. Early predictors of in-hospital mortality for Pneumocystis carinii pneumonia in acquired immunodeficiency síndrome. Arch Intern Med 1987;147:1413.

[52] McClellan MD, Millar SB, Parsons PE, Cohn DL, Pneumothorax with Pneumocystis carinii pneumonia in AIDS. Incidente and clinical characteristics. Chest 1991 100;1224-8.

[53] Tumbarello M, Tacconelli E, Pirronti T, et al. Pneumocystis carinii pneumonia and pulmonary tuberculosis. Eur Respir J 1997;10:1332-5.

[54] Ravinglione MC. Extrapulmonary pneumocystosis: the first 50 cases. Rev Infect Dis. 1990;12:1127-1138.

[55] Amin MB, Abrash MP, Mezger E, et al. Systemic dissemination of Pneumocystis carinii in a patient with acquired immunodeficiency síndrome. Henry Ford Hosp. Med J. 1990;38:68-71.

[56] Battan R, Mariuz P, Ravinglione MC, et al. Pneumocystis carinii infection of the thyroid in a hypothyroid patient with AIDS: diagnosis by fine leedle aspiration biopsy. J Clin Endocrinol Metab. 1991;72:724-726.

[57] Harris C, Specter B, Lim W. Unique chest radriograph features of CMV complicating PCP in HIV infected infants. Int Conf AIDS. 1993 Jun 6-11;9:360. (Abstract N PO-B08-1347)

[58] Castro J, Mansi G, Espinoza L, Campos M, Boulanger C. Concurrent PCP and TB Pneumonia in HIV Infected Patients. Scandinavian Journal of Infectious Diseases. 2007;39:1054-1058.

[59] Masur H, Shelhamer J. Empiric outpatient management of HIV-related pneumonia:economical or unwise? Ann Intern Med. 1996;124:451-453.

[60] Luce JM, Stover DE. Controversies in pulmonary medicine: presumed *Pneumocystis carinii* pneumonia should be treated in patients with the acquired immunodeficiency syndrome. Pro and con. Am Rev Respir Dis. 1988;138:1076-1077.

[61] Gruden JF, Huang L, Turner J, et al. High resolution CT in the evaluation of clinically suspected Pneumocystis carinii pneumonia in AIDS patients with normal, equivocal, or nospecific radiograph findings. Am J Roentgenol 1997;169:967.

[62] Tuazon CN, Delaney MD, Simm GL, et al. Utility of Gallium-67 scintigraphy and bronchial washing in the diagnosis of Pneumocystis carinii pneumonia in patients with the acquired immune deficiency syndrome. Am Rev Respir Dis 1985;132:1087.

[63] Stover DE, Meduri GU. Pulmonary function tests. Clin Chest Med. 1988;9:473.

[64] Phair J, Munoz A, Detels R, et al. The risk of Pneumocystis carinii pneumonia among men infected with the human immunodeficiency virus type I. Multicenter AIDS cohort study group. N Eng J Med 1990;322:161.

[65] Zaman MK, White DA. Serum lactate dehydrogenase levels and Pneumocystis carinii pneumonia: Diagnostic and prognostic significance. Am Rev Respir Dis 1988;137:796.

[66] Butt AA, Michaels S, Kissinger P. The association of serum lactate dehydrogenase level with selected opportunistic infections and HIV progression. Int J Infect Dis 2002;6:178.

[67] Quist J, Hill AR. Serum lactate dehydrogenase (LDH) in Pneumocystis carinii pneumonia, tuberculosis, and bacterial pneumonia. Chest 1995;108:415-8.

[68] Zaman MK, Wooten OJ, Suprahmanya B, et al. Rapid non-invasive diagnosis of Pneumocystis carinii from induced liquefied sputum. Ann Intern Med 1988;109-17.

[69] Cruciani M, Marcati P, Malena M, et al. Meta-analysis of diagnostic procedures for Pneumocystis carinii pneumonia in HIV-1 infected patients. Eur Respir J 2002;20:982.

[70] Willocks L, Burns S, Cossar R, Brettle R. Diagnosis of Pneumocystis carinii pneumonia in a population of HIV-positive drug users, with particular reference to sputum induction and fluorescent antibobies techniques. J Infect 1993;26:257.

[71] Bigby TD. Diagnosis of Pneumocystis carinii pneumonia: how invasive? Chest 1994;105:650-2.

[72] Armbruster C, Pokieser L, Hassl A. Diagnosis of Pneumocystis carinii pneumonia by bronchoalveolar lavage in AIDS patients: comparison of Diff-Quik, fungifluor stain, direct immunofluorescence test and polymerase chain reaction. Acta Cytol 1995;39:1089-93.

[73] Ortona E, Margutti P, de luca A, et al. Non specific PCR products using rat-derived Pneumocystis carinii dihydrofolate reductase gene-specific primers in DNA amplification of human respiratory samples. Mol Cell Probes 1996;10:187-90.

[74] Wakefield AE, Guiver L, Miller RF, Hopkin JM. DNA amplification on induced sputum samples for diagnosis of Pneumocystis carinii pneumonia. Lancet 1991;337:1378-9.

[75] Larsen HH, Masur H, Kovacs J, et al. Development and evaluation of a quantitative, touch-down, real-time PCR assay for diagnosing Pneumocystis carinii pneumonia. J Clin Microbiol 2002;40:490.

[76] Zingale A, Carrera P, Lazzarin A, Scarpellini P. Detection of Pneumocystis carinii and characterization of mutations associated with sulfa resistance in bronchoalveolar lavage samples from human immunodeficiency virus-infected subjects. J Clin Microbiol 2003;41:2709.

[77] Skelly M, Hoffman J, Fabbri M, et al. S-adenosylmethionine concentrations in diagnosis of Pneumocystis carinii pneumonia. Lancet 2003;361:1267-8.

[78] Safrin S, Finkelstein DM, Feinberg J, et al. Comparison of three regimens for treatment of mild to moderate Pneumocystis carinii pneumonia in patients with AIDS. Ann Intern Med 1996;124:792-802.

[79] Espinoza, LA. *Pneumocystis* Pneumonia. In HIV/AIDS Primary Care Guide. Beal J, Orrick JJ, Alfonso K, editors. Crown House Publishing Company LLC. 2006:355-8.

[80] Kessl J.J. et al. Molecular basis for atovaquone resistance in Pneumocystis jirovecii modeled in the cytochrome bc(1) complex of Saccharomyces cerevisiae. J Biol hem. 2004;279:2817-24.

[81] Consensus statement on the use of corticosteroids as adjunctive therapy for Pneumocystis pneumonia in the acquired immunodeficiency syndrome. N Engl J Med 1990;323:1500-4.

[82] Miller RF, Allen E, Copas A, et al. Improved survival for HIV infected patients with severe Pneumocystis jiroveci pneumonia is independent of highly active antiretroviral therapy. Thorax 2006; 61:716-721.

[83] Curtis JR, Yarnold PR, Schwartz DN, et al. Improvements in outcomes of acute respiratory failure for patients with human immunodeficiency virus-related Pneumocystis carinii pneumonia. Am J Resp Crit Care Med 2000; 162:393-8.

[84] Morris A, Creasman J, Turner J, et al. Intensive care of human immunodeficiency virus-infected patients during the era of highly antiretroviral therapy. Am J Resp Crit Care Med 2002; 166:262-7.

[85] Yale SH, Limper AH. *Pneumocystis carinii* pneumonia in patients without acquired immunodeficiency syndrome: associated illness and prior corticosteroid therapy. Mayo Clin Proc 1996;71:5-13.

[86] Curtis JR, Yarnold PR, Schwartz DN, et al. Improvements in outcomes of acute respiratory failure for patients with human immunodeficiency virus-related Pneumocystis carinii pneumonia. Am J Resp Crit Care Med 2000; 162:393-8.

[87] Crothers K, Beard CB, Turner J, et al. Severity and outcome of HIV-associated Pneumocystis pneumonia containing Pneumocystis jiroveci dihydropteroate Synthase gene mutations. AIDS 2005;19:801-5.

In: AIDS- Related Opportunistic Infections
Editor: Claudia D. Galanda

ISBN: 978-1-60692-144-9

Chapter IV

On the Finding of Trichomonads as Co-Infecting Agents in *Pneumocystis* Pneumonia

Christophe Duboucher,[1] Eduardo Dei-Cas[2] and Eric Viscogliosi[3]

[1] Department of Pathology, Poissy/Saint-Germain Hospital
Saint-Germain-en-Laye, France

[2] Department of Ecology of Parasitism, Lille Pasteur Institute and
Lille 2 University Hospital Centre, Lille, France

[3] Lille Pasteur Institute and Lille 2 University, Lille, France

Abstract

In recent years, we have observed that *Pneumocystis* pneumonia (PcP) is frequently super-infected by trichomonads, whereas PcP was thought to be a single opportunistic infection caused by *Pneumocystis jirovecii.* Moreover, in cases rich in *Pneumocystis* organisms, the frequency of coinfection with trichomonads in alveoli can reach 100%. On the other hand, we have observed that super-infection by trichomonads could develop as well in immunocompetent patients, for instance in the course of acute respiratory distress syndrome (ARDS). This latter finding reinforces the view that in PcP trichomonads express a peculiar form of opportunism, where local conditions in alveolar lumens play a major role instead of immunodeficiency. Trichomonads development could be a secondary event in alveoli filled by *Pneumocystis*, and eradication of the fungus should therefore be followed by elimination of protists. Thus, these data could not have implications in patient management. However, they raise many questions in several fields that are examined in this Commentary: a) questions about the delay of such a report since the start of the AIDS epidemic, b) questions about the source of trichomonads and species involved, and c) questions about the role of trichomonads in PcP and their potential deleterious effect. Data about trichomonads found in the course of PcP are mainly observational. Nevertheless, currently proposed pathophysiological

Corresponding author: Dr. Duboucher, Poissy/Saint-Germain Hospital, Department of Pathology, 20 Rue Armagis, 78100 Saint-Germain-en-laye, France .christophe.duboucher@online.fr. Tel: +33.1.39.27.42.10 Fax: +33.1. 39.27.42.14

conceptions of PcP could be reconsidered in the future at the levels of both clinical and biological research.

Introduction

Until recently, *Pneumocystis* pneumonia (PcP) was thought to be a single opportunistic infection caused by the fungus *Pneumocystis jirovecii*. For the last years, we have observed that PcP patients are frequently super-infected by trichomonads in their lungs, and that the rate of co-infection reach 100% when *Pneumocystis* organisms burden the alveoli, allowing us to hypothesize the so-called PcP disease results from co-infection. However, until now, this co-infection has not been proclaimed. This situation raises many questions that are discussed in this commentary dealing with the biology of trichomonads and *Pneumocystis*, a way of detection used by observers – mainly parasitologists and cytopathologists – and epistemological considerations.

1. On the Discovery of Co-Infection of *Pneumocystis* Pneumonia by Trichomonads.

In 2002, a bronchoalveolar lavage fluid (BALF) sample was sent to the Saint-Germain-en-Laye Hospital Pathology laboratory (France) [1]. The explored patient was a 41-year-old black man, presented with fever, increasing dyspnea and extensive ground glass opacities. Unknown infection by human immunodeficiency virus (HIV-1) was revealed by laboratory tests and *Pneumocystis* pneumonia (PcP) was confirmed by detecting numerous cysts of *Pneumocystis* sp. Searches for *Toxoplasma* and nuclear inclusions of cytomegalovirus or Herpes type viruses by standard examination and immuno-histochemistry were negative in the BALF sample, as was the search for acid-fast bacilli. Surprisingly, numerous cells that are not usually observed in BALFs were found on the slide routinely stained with May-Grünwald-Giemsa (MGG). These cells showed salient polymorphism but there were always transition forms indicating a common nature. Elsewhere, nuclear characteristics were not those of human cells and a parasite – a protist – was evoked. These cells were also found on MGG stained cytospins processed in the microbiology laboratory where another sample of the BALF had been sent. A contaminant from a coloration bath, such as infusoria growing in old reagents, was then absolutely excluded. Morphological characteristics of numerous cells were similar to those observed in two cases of trichomonoses of head and neck region published in recent years by the same observer [2, 3]. Lastly, characteristics were quite different from those of other protists observed in humans such as amoeba or *Giardia lamblia*. Infestation by a trichomonad or a related parasite was the final conclusion and an exact identification was performed using molecular tools. By small subunit (SSU) rRNA gene amplification followed by sequencing, the protist was identified as *Trichomonas vaginalis* (*T. vaginalis*) [1]. The SSU ribosomal rRNA gene is the most used marker in molecular phylogeny at the species level. It is the most sequenced gene and sequences of numerous animals, plants, and fungi are available. Thus, this sequence is also used for identification by PCR or detection by *in situ* hybridization, in many fields of biology or parasitology, and in human pathology as well as in veterinary pathology.

At that time, this case of co-infection by *Pneumocystis* sp. and *T. vaginalis* was believed to be isolated, but it was not very amazing in regard to our experience with other sites. Some months later, the discovery of the same parasitic cells in another newly obtained BALF sample from a PcP patient incited us to search for these parasites retrospectively in stored BALF samples of former patients. Trichomonads were found as coinfecting agents in 60% of the BALF samples of patients diseased from PcP [4]. More, abundance of trichomonads increased in the cases with highest *Pneumocystis* rates, and frequency reached 100%. This fact, considered alone, could result from better fibroscopic collecting, without indication of the exact location of parasites. However, trichomonads were found whatever the level of contamination by pharyngeal or bronchial cells, indicating that the protist came from alveolar lumen together with the fungus *Pneumocystis*. Thus, this high frequency of co-infection suggests that the lung disease called PcP may be considered as a pulmonary co-infection by *Pneumocystis* and trichomonads.

2. On the Significance of Such Colonization

What is the reason of such a co-infection ? The presence of trichomonads in BALF of PcP patients shows that these protists are able to grow in the alveolar lumen. In AIDS patients without obvious lung disease, in whom BAL was performed to explore unexplained fever, trichomonads are not found. Thus, the growing of *Pneumocystis* seems to be a critical condition to the development of trichomonads in lung alveoli. One hypothesis is that trichomonads fed on fungus. The ability of *T. vaginalis* for phagocytosis and degradation of the fungus *Saccharomyces cerevisiae* has been well described [5]. By optical microscopy on cytospins of BALF samples from PcP patients, tight contacts between trichomonads and *Pneumocystis* aggregates or isolated trophozoites are observed, but further ultrastructural analysis is required. A second hypothesis – which is not opposite to the first one – is that trichomonads development is promoted by another condition. Trichomonads are microaerophilic organisms that tolerate only lower levels of oxygen [6, 7]. Reduction of ventilation generated by *Pneumocystis* pullulating may create the environment poor in oxygen required for trichomonad development.

An important finding that has reinforced this point of view was the observation of trichomonads in BALF samples from patients with non-PcP pulmonary diseases. Actually, we detected trichomonads also in BALF samples from patients presenting with ARDS [8]. In these patients, super-infection by trichomonads was not correlated with any trait, such as age, immunodepression, associated disease, other infections, antibiotic or corticosteroid treatments. The sole factor that differentiated patients with or without trichomonads was the day of BALF sampling. Indeed, in trichomonad-infected patients, BAL was carried out later. These findings reinforce the opinion that trichomonads infection in both conditions – PcP and ARDS – is not mainly linked to immunodepression, but to a local and specific environment in alveolar lumens. In these situations, the local conditions observed are *Pneumocystis* burden in

PcP, and a diffuse alveolar damage in ARDS. In the late phases of diffuse alveolar damage – morphologic substratum of ARDS – after the initial exsudative phase, alveolar lumens are filled by hyaline membranes and cell debris. As in PcP, ventilation is reduced, creating an environment poor in oxygen that is required for the development of the microaerophilic trichomonads. To resume, trichomonads development is a secondary event, occurring once favorable local conditions are created, and could be a potential event in all patients developing *Pneumocystis* infection.

3. On the Occultation of Trichomonads

The crucial question that everybody wonders is the reason for so long a delay to report this co-infection, whereas tens of thousands of BALF samples from PcP patients have been screened since the start of the AIDS epidemic. In our opinion, the first and main reason is that, in the BALF of these patients, trichomonads do not exhibit the classical free ovoid form, i.e., the flagellated form that is well known by parasitologists. Flagellated form is only one of the avatars of this protist; another avatar is the amoeboid form. Indeed, transformation of flagellated into amoeboid forms is a characteristic of trichomonads. These cells are able to develop pseudopods *in vitro* when adhering to coverslips [9] or to host cells in culture systems [10] or *in vivo* when adhering to vaginal epithelial cells [11]. A dense network of actin-rich microfilaments is observed by electron microscopy along the adhesion zone [11]. Transformation to amoeboid forms involves reduction of microtubular structures (flagella and axostyle-pelta complex) as such structures were not detected by light microscopy in BALF cytospin slides stained with MGG, or by immuno-cytochemistry using a specific anti-tubulin monoclonal antibody [1]. Trichomonads present in lungs in amoeboid form, i.e., as an anonymous cell that has lost its distinctive mark and that mimics a human cell.

Two groups of observers can be facing trichomonads: parasitologists and cytopathologists. In fresh specimens – vaginal secretions or urines – parasitologists detect currently trichomonads that present in flagellated form. They recognize parasites by the motion of their flagella. On a cytological slide, dried and stained by MGG, these flagellated forms remain recognizable. Flagella, axostyle-pelta complex and parabasal apparatus are well visible. On the other hand, in BALF samples, where trichomonads coming from alveolar lumens are in amoeboid form, there is no more way to recognize the protist by the above criteria in fresh specimen, as well as on MGG stained cytospins. Therefore, it is not surprising that trichomonads have not been noticed by parasitologists in BALF samples of PcP patients. When a BALF sample is collected by fibroscopy, a part is currently sent to a cytopathology laboratory for cell counting and detection of atypical cells. The field of experience of cytopathologists is human cells, especially cells that are found in BALF in normal or pathological conditions: alveolar macrophages, inflammatory cells, desquamation of epithelial cells and tumoral cells. Thus, amoeboid trichomonads can catch the eye of the observer because they don't fall into one category of normal or tumoral cells. The observer can recognize these “alien” cells and can declare them as "parasitic protists" without being wrong. Thus, a question that is raised here is why the cytopathologist cannot say more, even though he regularly observes trichomonads in vaginal smears ? Vaginal smears are colored by the Papanicolaou's stain, because observation of epithelial cells is prioritized. The appearance of trichomonads colored by Papanicolaou's stain is quite different from that of trichomonads colored by MGG. It must be said that in Pap smears trichomonads are not recognized by their flagella – not stained – but by their calibrated shape and their faintly stained elliptic nucleus. What is recognized by the cytopathologist in Pap smears is not a flagellated parasite but a kind of cell ghost that is declared "trichomonad" without risk of error (Figure 1, A & B).

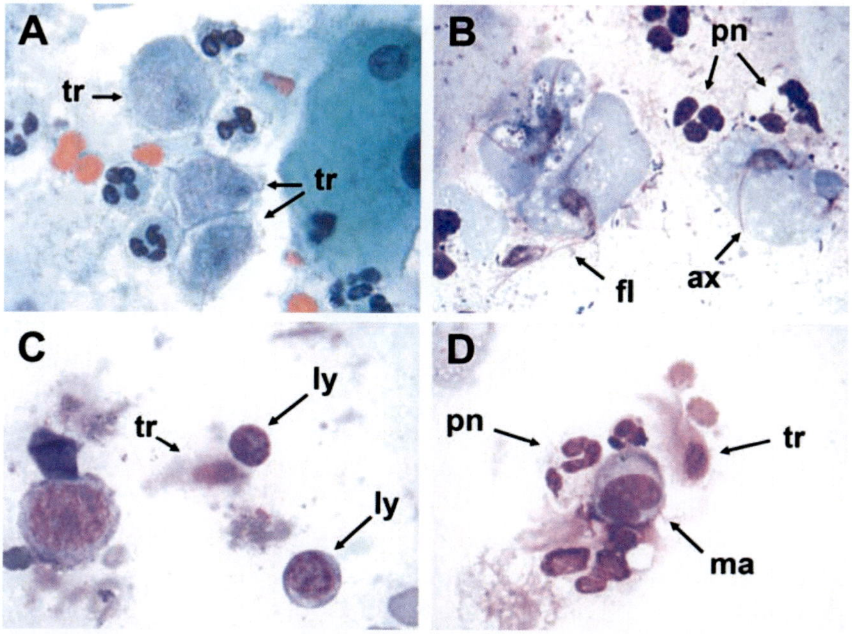

A *Trichomonas vaginalis* in a vaginal smear (Papanicolaou's stain; x 1000). **B** *Trichomonas vaginalis* in a vaginal smear (MGG; x 1000). **C** *Trichomonas tenax* in a lymph node (MGG; x 1000). **D** *Trichomonas vaginalis* in a case of pneumocystosis (MGG; x 1000). Arrows indicate trichomonads (tr), axostyle (ax), flagella (fl), neutrophils (pn), lymphocytes (ly), and, macrophagic cells (ma).

Figure 1. - Morphological aspects of trichomonads under different conditions of observation.

Commentaries on Figure 1

A. This microphotograph shows what is seen by cytopathologists in a vaginal smear colored by Papanicolaou's stain. This stain is well adapted to malpighian epithelial cells, and allows discovery of atypical cells. Trichomonads, *T. vaginalis*, are recognizable by their small ovoid and faintly colored nucleus. Trichomonads are identified by their overall appearance, and not by other structures – parabasal body, flagella and axostyle – which are not visible.

B. This microphotograph shows the same cells in a vaginal smear, but colored by MGG. MGG stain, used for hematological spreads, is not suitable for malpighian epithelial cells, and is not used in cervico-vaginal screening. This coloration shows perfectly that numerous trichomonad cells are flagellated. Parabasal body, flagella (fl) and axostyle (ax) are well visible. Trichomonad cells in amoeboid form, which lack these identification structures, are normally present, but are not distinguishable from small epithelial cells. Existence of amoeboid forms, the form adopted by the parasite when adhering to epithelial cells, is nevertheless confirmed by electron microscopy [11].

Figures 1A and 1B show *T. vaginalis* at the same magnification and from the same patient. Contrarily to Papanicolaou's stain, MGG stain is not preceded by fixation. In Fig 1B, the cell is well laid out, as a fried egg, and in Fig. 1A the cell is congealed as a boiled egg. Different aspects of the nucleus are striking.

C. *Trichomonas tenax* in a lymph node. This slide is a touch print of a freshly cut lymph node. By this procedure, mechanical artifacts are excluded. The parasitic cells exhibit no structure such as parabasal body, flagella or axostyle. This is the ideal appearance of the amoeboid form of a trichomonad, sampled and colored in the best conditions.

D. *Trichomonas vaginalis* in a broncho alveolar lavage fluid. As in Fig. 1C, no structure is visible within the body, nor flagella at the top of the cell. The parasite has involuted into an anonymous cell, which nevertheless contrasts with the human cells present in the lavage. These cells that are not of human origin can attract the eye of the cytopathologist, who is trained to the analysis of human cells.

As said above, even though MGG stain is used on cytospsins of BALF, which is the best routine stain to observe these cells in biological specimens, structures that could give the "key" have disappeared in amoeboid cells. Moreover, facing the "alien" cells that the cytopathologist has claimed "unidentified parasite", this cytopathologist cannot be supported by a parasitologist for the same reason (Figure 1, C & D).

Other reasons for the occultation of trichomonads in PCP refer to the observer rather than to the misleading morphology of trichomonads. Away from the genito-urinary tract, and facing a trichomonad in BALF that has developed into an amoeboid form, nobody – neither parasitologists nor cytopathologists – is ready to consider trichomonads in this location. Moreover, almost all observers recognizing trichomonads by their flagella are unaware of amoeboid forms. The traditional taxonomic position of trichomonads as "flagellates" has led to the erroneous conception that trichomonads always bear flagella. Yet lack of flagella does not exclude trichomonad. By the above cited observations [2, 3], we have the experience of this misleading presentation of amoeboid trichomonads that gave us the "key". Trichomonads co-infecting PcP patients became an expected event after this experience.

These commentaries should explain why the presence of trichomonads associated with *Pneumocystis* has not been reported until recently. It is perhaps here the price of the progress. Extent of knowledge has led to overspecialization and to a detrimental division of specialities. One observer – the cytopathologist – recognizes a parasitic cell because it does not look like a human cell. The other one – the parasitologist – who has the competence to identify parasites, does it by comparison with reference pictures of parasites. It is not surprising that a known parasite in an unknown form has remained overlooked until now. It is a real paradox that these parasitic cells, the size of which is that of a small human cell, and which are visible through a simple optical microscope, have not been remarked in BALFs of PcP during the last decades. For many of us, progress in microbiology walk concurrently with increasing resolution of observation. Electron microscopy and molecular biology have propelled us to the molecular level. Advances in understanding pathogenesis of PcP are at the molecular level [12]. Nevertheless, dealing with PcP, we can also gain by moving back. Cytopathologists, when examining BALFs, look for tumor cells. They work in another scale of magnification and another field than microbiologists. The higher magnification used by the first ones is a low magnification for the second ones. Examination of a BALF of PcP at low magnification, with detachment, allows us to appraise cellular composition. The eye of a cytopathologist alone, who is trained to analyze human cells, can be attracted by cells that are frequently found in PcP and that are not human cells (Figure 2, A to D). To resume, our findings are not resulting from the search of a parasite, but from identification of anonymous cells mimicking human cells in the cellular environment of PcP.

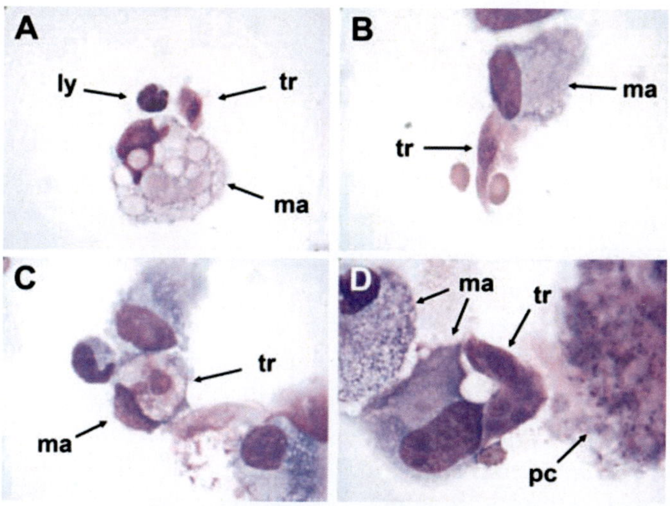

Different forms found in a broncho alveolar lavage fluid of a patient diseased from *Pneumocystis* pneumonia are presented (MGG; x 1000): a small form (**A**), a larger form (**B**), a form lying flat on a macrophagic cell (or engulfed in ?) (**C**), and a trinucleated form (**D**).

Arrows indicate trichomonads (tr), macrophagic cells (ma), lymphocytes (ly), and pneumocystis (pc).

To illustrate completely this Commentary, we have also included on a web site a large number of microphotographs from other samples, collected in various situations including PcP and in different institutions (http://www.trichomonosis.net/).

Figure 2. - Amoeboid trichomonads observed during co-infection with *Pneumocystis*

4. On the Species Involved

Until recently, the presence of trichomonads in the human respiratory tract was considered a rare occurrence. That was reported mostly in patients with underlying pulmonary diseases [13]. The parasite was often identified as *Trichomonas tenax* (*T. tenax*), a saprophyte found in the mouth. Nevertheless, *T. vaginalis* has been isolated from lungs in cases of neonatal infection [14].

Identification of species is classically based on morphological criteria visible through an optical microscope, such as the number of anterior flagella, the morphology of parabasal apparatus and the axostyle-pelta complex. As stated above, these structures are missing in amoeboid forms. In the first case report of co-infection by a trichomonad and *Pneumocystis* sp., we have performed identification by molecular way. By amplification of the SSU rRNA gene followed by sequencing, we could identify the species as *T. vaginalis* [1]. It was both amazing and not amazing. On the one hand, the four trichomonads found in humans are considered as site specific (i.e. organ specific) [15]: *T. tenax* in the oral cavity, *T. vaginalis* in the genitourinary tract, and *Pentatrichomonas hominis* and *Dientamoeba fragilis* in the intestinal tract. On the other hand, *T. vaginalis* has been found in lungs during neonatal infections [14], in a case of oesophageal trichomoniasis in an HIV-negative immunodeficient patient [16], and in pharyngeal specimens of HIV-positive men with history of orogenital activity [17]. In another case of co-infection, the amplification of the Internal Transcribed spacer 1 (ITS1)-5.8S rRNA-ITS2 region followed by sequencing, allowed us to identify the species *Tritrichomonas foetus* (*T. foetus*) [18]. *T. foetus* is a pathogen of the bovine reproductive tract and causes infertility and spontaneous abortions. Close related species, which cannot be distinguished by molecular tools alone, are found in pigs (known as *Tritrichomonas suis*), cats, and monkeys (known as *Tritrichomonas mobilensis*). This case could be interpreted as a zoonotic infection transmitted from one of the natural hosts of *Tritrichomonas* species. Nevertheless, at the same time, two strains of the genus *Tetratrichomonas* were isolated by others, from the respiratory tract of humans [19], which exhibited a close genetic relationship with the avian species *Tetratrichomonas gallinarum*. The same authors failed to transmit *Tetratrichomonas* of human origin to birds. That fact may be explained by a biological separation of the human-host-adapted *T. gallinarum*-like trichomonads from the genuine *T. gallinarum*. A similar explanation could be put forward in our case report, with the existence of a human-host-adapted *T. foetus*-like strain. The identification of two unexpected species of trichomonads co-infecting PcP – *T. vaginalis* and *T. foetus* – lets us believe that in the future, a more extensive examination of trichomonads found in lungs may reveal unexpected or unknown species, rather than *T. tenax*, the unique trichomonad known to inhabit oral cavity [13]. A protist is considered saprophyte, as long as a pathogen effect has not been observed. Perhaps, when local conditions become favorable – such as in PcP – unknown or known species of trichomonads, which inhabit niches as saprophytes, may proliferate. Systematic (or almost) occurrence of co-infection by trichomonads argues for this conception. Zoonotic species, which don't settle regularly in humans, may also find here conditions for their development. Contrarily to obvious pathogens, saprophyte organisms – bacteria, protists or fungi – present usually a limited interest to medical researchers. In so far as they are not identified as pathogenic, saprophyte organisms are not targeted by biomedical research. *Helicobacter pylori* is a striking illustration [20]. AIDS offers local conditions – PcP and other opportunistic infections – combined to general condition – deep immunodepression – that may favor the proliferation of such saprophytes, which may remain overlooked as long as they are not identified.

5. On the Deleterious Action and on the Treatment

Other important issues concern the potential pathogenic role of trichomonads in the lungs and anti-trichomonad drug administering. The principal fact that argues against harmlessness of trichomonads is their amoeboid transformation, which is enhanced by contact with target cells and reinforces adhesion. After this contact, different genes are upregulated in *T. vaginalis*, inducing adhesin and α-actinin syntheses [21]. Such amoeboid forms of *T. vaginalis* are able *in vitro* to induce deleterious effects on epithelial cells [22, 23]. For instance; it has been shown that *T. foetus* and *T. vaginalis* induce apoptosis of epithelial and macrophagic cells [24-27]. Thus, amoeboid transformation is the hallmark of adhesion to host cells and aggressive behavior of trichomonad cells.

In BALF samples from PcP patients, trichomonads in amoeboid form are frequently observed in close contact with alveolar macrophages. Moreover, phagocytosis and the degradation of parasitic cells were observed in several BALF specimens, indicating that macrophages play an active role in host defense against trichomonads. The adhesion of trichomonads to epithelial cells was not observed but alveolar epithelial cells are usually rare in BALF samples, as these cells are strongly attached to the basement membrane. In the context of diffuse alveolar damage, the epithelial layer is destroyed and only a few dystrophic alveolar epithelial cells are observed. The interaction of trichomonads with alveolar epithelial cells cannot be visualized in BALF samples, and requires *in vitro* models, such as the co-culture of alveolar epithelial cells and trichomonads, or lung biopsies from PcP patients suitable for ultrastructural studies. There is another fact that can be evoked to argue for a deleterious effect of trichomonads. Indeed, two trichomonad species have been identified in BALF of PcP i. e. *T. vaginalis* and *T. foetus*. It is noteworthy that these two species are recognized as pathogens either in humans (*T. vaginalis*) or in cattle (*T. foetus*) [28].

All these data strongly suggest that trichomonads can play a deleterious effect role in alveolar lumen. Thus, administering a treatment against these protists should be considered. PcP healing results from the elimination of *Pneumocystis* with appropriated drugs, even though trimethoprime-sulfamethoxazole (TMP-SMX) is not active against *T. vaginalis*, and probably against other trichomonads [29]. As discussed above, it appears that trichomonads settlement in alveolar lumens is a secondary event promoted by *Pneumocystis* multiplication and other local conditions. Restitution of original conditions in alveolar lumen would be followed by the disappearance of the protist. Even though PcP is a more complex disease than a simple infection by the fungus *Pneumocystis*, it could be believed that the ending of the triggering factor – that is *Pneumocystis* – is sufficient to cure PcP. Nevertheless, in severe forms of PcP, when diffuse alveolar damage is combined, trichomonads could persist in alveolar lumen although eradication of the fungus has been obtained by TMP-SMX. In these cases, as in ARDS of any origin, it is not excluded that trichomonads may act in the delay of healing and limitation of recovery [8].

Conclusion

Even though some contributions have been published to the comprehension of the co-infection *Pneumocystis*-trichomonads, many questions remain unanswered. Some facts are sound such as the development of trichomonads as a secondary event that occurs almost always with time in the course of PcP and ARDS. Moreover, the deleterious action of trichomonads in alveoli is suggested through different observations but remains to be confirmed. In addition, the infection source and spectrum of trichomonads species able to invade human lungs will be clarified in the further studies. Beyond what is brought to comprehension of PcP, co-infection with trichomonads recalls that many things remain to be discovered in medicine and science obviously by studies in-depth and by powerful tools. In some cases, we shall gain in watching with naive eyes what others have neglected, in studying observations without narrow-mindedness, or in questioning what is sententiously taught. No clue must be neglected, as in a detective fiction, even though appearances seem enough [30].

References

[1] Duboucher, C; Noël, C; Durand-Joly, I; Gerbod, D; Delgado-Viscogliosi, P; Jouveshomme, S; Leclerc, C; Cartolano, G-L; Dei-Cas, E; Capron, M; Viscogliosi, E. Pulmonary co-infection by *Trichomonas vaginalis* and *Pneumocystis* sp. as a novel manifestation of AIDS. *Hum Pathol*, 2003 34, 508-511.

[2] Duboucher, C; Mogenet, M; Périé, G. Salivary trichomoniasis; a case report of infestation of a submaxillary gland by *Trichomonas tenax*. *Arch Pathol Lab Med*, 1995 119, 277-279.

[3] Duboucher, C; Farto-Bensasson, F; Chéron, M; Peltier, J-Y; Beaufils, F; Périé, G. Lymph node infection by *Trichomonas tenax*: report of a case with co-infection by *Mycobacterium tuberculosis*. *Human Pathol*, 2000 31, 1317-1321.

[4] Duboucher, C; Gerbod, D; Noël, C; Durand-Joly, I; Delgado-Viscogliosi, P; Leclerc, C; Pham, S; Capron, M; Dei-Cas, E; Viscogliosi, E. Frequency of trichomonads as coinfecting agents in *Pneumocystis* pneumonia. *Acta Cytol*, 2005 49, 273-277.

[5] Pereira-Neves, A; Benchimol, M. Phagocytosis by *Trichomonas vaginalis*: new insights. *Biol Cell*, 2007 99, 87-101.

[6] Ellis, JE; Cole, D; Lloyd, D. Influence of oxygen on the fermentative metabolism of metronidazole-sensitive and resistant strains of *Trichomonas vaginalis*. *Mol Biochem Parasitol*, 1992 56, 79-88.

[7] Ellis, JE; Yarlett, N; Cole, D; Humphreys, MJ; Lloyd, D. Antioxidant defences in the microaerophilic protozoan *Trichomonas vaginalis*: comparison of metronidazole-resistant and sensitive strains. *Microbiology*, 1994 140, 2489-2494.

[8] Duboucher, C; Barbier, C; Beltramini, A; Rona, M; Ricome, J-L; Morel, G; Capron, M; Pierce, RJ; Dei-Cas, E; Viscogliosi, E. Pulmonary superinfection by trichomonads in the course of Acute Respiratory Distress Syndrome. *Lung*, 2007 185, 295-301.

[9] Brugerolle, G; Bricheux, G; Coffe, G. Actin cytoskeleton demonstration in *Trichomonas vaginalis* and in other trichomonads. *Biol Cell*, 1996 88, 29-36.

[10] Arroyo, R; Gonzalez-Robles, A; Martinez-Palomo, A; Alderete, JF. Signalling of *Trichomonas vaginalis* for amoeboid transformation and adhesion synthesis follows cytoadherence. *Mol Microbiol*, 1993 7, 299-309.

[11] Nielsen, MH; Nielsen, R. Electron microscopy of *Trichomonas vaginalis* Donné: interaction with vaginal epithelium in human trichomoniasis. *Acta Pathol Microbiol Scand [B]*, 1975 83, 305-320.

[12] Thomas, CF Jr; Limper, AH. Current insights into the biology and pathogenesis of *Pneumocystis* pneumonia. *Nat Rev Microbiol*, 2007 5, 298-308.

[13] Hersh, SM. Pulmonary trichomoniasis and *Trichomonas tenax*. *J Med Microbiol*, 1985 20, 1-10.

[14] Carter, JE; Whithaus, KC. Neonatal respiratory tract involvement by *Trichomonas vaginalis*: a case report and review of the literature. *Am J Trop Med Hyg*, 2008 78, 17-19.

[15] Honigberg, BM. Trichomonads found outside the urogenital tract of humans, 342-393. *In* Trichomonads Parasitic in Humans. Honigberg BM. New York, NY. Springer-Verlag; 1990.

[16] Guccion, JG; Ortega, LG. Trichomoniasis complicating esophageal intramural pseudodiverticulosis: diagnosis by transmission electron microscopy. *Ultrastruct Pathol*, 1996 20, 101-107.

[17] Press, N; Chavez, VM; Ticona, E; Calderon, M; Apolinario, IS; Culotta, A; Arevalo, J; Gilman, RH; Working Group on AIDS in Peru. Screening for sexually transmitted diseases in human immunodeficiency virus-positive patients in Peru reveals an absence of *Chlamydia trachomatis* and identifies *Trichomonas vaginalis* in pharyngeal specimens. *Clin Infect Dis*, 2001 32, 808-814.

[18] Duboucher, C; Caby, S; Dufernez, F; Chabé, M; Gantois, N; Delgado-Viscogliosi, P; Billy, C; Barré, E; Torabi, E; Capron, M; Pierce, RJ; Dei-Cas, E; Viscogliosi, E. Molecular identification of *Tritrichomonas foetus*-like organisms as coinfecting agents of human *Pneumocystis* pneumonia. *J Clin Microbiol*, 2006 44, 1165-1168.

[19] Kutisova, K; Kulda, J; Cepicka, I; Flegr, J; Koudela, B; Teras, J; Tachezy, J. Tetratrichomonads from the oral cavity and respiratory tract of humans. *Parasitology*, 2005 131, 1-11.

[20] Marshall, BJ; Warren, JR. Unidentified curved bacilli in the stomach of patients with gastritis and peptic ulceration. *Lancet*, 1984 1, 1311-1315.

[21] Kucknoor, AS; Mundodi, V; Alderete, JF. Adherence to human vaginal epithelial cells signals for increased expression of *Trichomonas vaginalis* genes. *Infect Immun*, 2005 73, 6472-6478.

[22] Jesus, JB; Vannier-Santos, MA; Britto, C; Godefroy, P; Silva-Filho, FC; Pinheiro, AA; Rocha-Azevedo, B; Lopes, AH; Meyer-Fernandes, JR. *Trichomonas vaginalis* virulence against epithelial cells and morphological variability: the comparison between a well-established strain and a fresh isolate. *Parasitol Res*, 2004 93, 369-377.

[23] Arroyo, R; Gonzalez-Robles, A; Martinez-Palomo, A; Alderete, JF. Signalling of *Trichomonas vaginalis* for amoeboid transformation and adhesion synthesis follows cytoadherence. *Mol Microbiol*, 1993 7, 299-309.

[24] Kucknoor, AS; Mundodi, V; Alderete, JF. *Trichomonas vaginalis* adherence mediates differential gene expression in human vaginal epithelial cells. *Cell Microbiol*, 2005 7, 887-897.

[25] Singh, BN; Lucas, JJ; Hayes GR; Kumar, I; Beach, DH; Frajblat, M; Gilbert, RO; Sommer, U; Costello, CE. *Tritrichomonas foetus* induces apoptotic cell death in bovine vaginal epithelial cells. *Infect Immun*, 2004 72, 4151-4158.

[26] Sommer, U; Costello, CE; Hayes, GR; Beach, DH; Gilbert, RO; Lucas, JJ; Singh, BN. Identification of *Trichomonas vaginalis* cysteine proteases that induce apoptosis in human vaginal epithelial cells. *J Biol Chem*, 2005 280, 23853-23860.

[27] Chang, JH; Kim, SK; Choi, IH; Lee, SK; Morio, T; Chang, EJ. Apoptosis of macrophages induced by *Trichomonas vaginalis* through the phosphorylation of p38 mitogen-activated protein kinase that locates at downstream of mitochondria-dependent caspase activation. *Int J Biochem Cell Biol*, 2006 38, 638-647.

[28] BonDurant, RH; Honigberg, BM. Trichomonads of veterinary importance, 111-188. *In* Parasitic protozoa, vol 9. 2nd ed. Kreier JP. New York, NY. Academic Press; 1994.

[29] Malagoli, M; Rossi, T; Baggio, A; Zandomeneghi, G; Zanca, A; Casolari, C; Castelli, M. "In vitro" study of chemotherapeutic activity of sulphimidazole on some sensitive and metronidazole-resistant *Trichomonas vaginalis* strains. *Pharmacol Res*, 2002 46, 469-472.

[30] Duboucher, C; Boggia, R; Morel, G; Capron, M; Pierce, RJ; Dei-Cas, E; Viscogliosi, E. *Pneumocystis* pneumonia: immunodepression, *Pneumocystis jirovecii*… and the third man. *Nat Rev Microbiol*, 2007 5, doi:10.1038/nrmicro1621-c1.

In: AIDS- Related Opportunistic Infections
Editor: Claudia D. Galanda

ISBN: 978-1-60692-144-9

Chapter V

AIDS-Related Opportunistic Infections in Children with Human Immunodeficiency Virus in the Era of Antiretroviral Therapy

***Danaya Chansinghakul*[1], *Thanyawee Puthanakit*[2] and *Chitsanu Pancharoen*[3]**

[1]Armed Forces Research Institute of Medical Sciences (AFRIMS), US Army Medical Component, Bangkok, Thailand

[2]HIV-NAT, The Thai Red Cross AIDS Research Center, Bangkok, Thailand

[3]Department of Pediatrics, Faculty of Medicine, Chulalongkorn University, Bangkok, Thailand

HIV-infected children are susceptible to opportunistic infections (OIs) due to immune suppression stage caused by HIV. Before the availability of antiretroviral therapy (ART), the common OIs among children were serious bacterial infections, *Pneumocystis jiroveci* pneumonia (PCP), candidiasis, herpes zoster, tuberculosis, disseminated *Mycobacterium avium* complex (MAC), and systemic fungal infection. Antiretroviral drugs control HIV viral replication and restore immune function. In the era of antiretroviral therapy, there is a significant reduction in rate of OIs which leads to reduction of morbidity and mortality in HIV-infected children. After HIV-infected children gain CD4 cell recovery while receiving stable antiretroviral therapy, opportunistic infection prophylaxis such as cotrimoxazole for PCP prophylaxis can be discontinued safely. In this article the perspectives of opportunistic infections management including immune reconstitution inflammatory syndrome and when to discontinue prophylaxis in the era of active antiretroviral therapy will be described.

Common AIDS-Related Opportunistic Infections in Pediatric HIV

In the pre-antiretroviral era and prior to the development of potent combination highly active antiretroviral treatment (HAART) regimens, opportunistic infections (OIs) were the primary cause of death in human immunodeficiency virus (HIV)-infected children [1]. However, few data are available regarding the overall prevalence, incidence and immunologic correlates associated with these diseases in the pediatric HIV population.

The natural history of OIs among children might differ from that observed among HIV-infected adults. Many OIs in adults are secondary to reactivation of opportunistic pathogens, which were often acquired before HIV infection at a time when host immunity was intact. However, OIs among HIV-infected children more often reflect primary infection with the pathogen and, among children with perinatal HIV infection, infection acquired after HIV infection has been established and begun to compromise an already immature immune system [2]. Without antiretroviral therapy, children who have been infected vertically with HIV progress from initial HIV infection to clinical AIDS at different rates and follow the bimodal pattern of clinical course: a smaller group of children develop AIDS rapidly and die within the first 1-2 years of life, and a larger group of children develop AIDS at slower rates that are closer to the rates seen in adults [3]. Some children who have been infected at birth have AIDS related symptoms and signs at 10 years of age or more [4].

The Pediatric AIDS Clinical Trials Group (PACTG) has conducted multicenter studies in HIV-positive children during the pre-HAART era since 1988 to determine the prevalence, event rates of various infectious complications and the immunologic correlates, specifically CD4 cell counts, associated with AIDS-related OIs [1]. The frequency of different opportunistic pathogens among HIV-infected children in the pre-HAART era varies with age, pathogen, prior OI and immunologic status. The most common initial OIs in children at event rates of >1.0 per 100 child-years (person years) were serious bacterial infections (with pneumonia, often presumptively diagnosed, and bacteremia being most common), herpes zoster, disseminated *Mycobacterium avium* complex (DMAC), *Pneumocystis jerovecii* pneumonia (PCP), and tracheobronchial and esophageal candidiasis. Less commonly observed OIs at event rate < 1.0 per 100 child-years included cytomegalovirus (CMV) disease, cryptosporidiosis, tuberculosis (TB), systemic fungal infections, and toxoplasmosis [5,6]. History of a previous AIDS-defining OI was a predictor of developing a new infection. Although the majority of infections occurred among children who were substantially immunocompromised, serious bacterial infections, herpes zoster, and TB occurred across the spectrum of immune status [7].

The details about the epidemiology, clinical presentation, diagnosis, treatment, and prophylaxis recommendations for each opportunistic pathogen are reviewed by the working group from Centers for Disease Control and Prevention, the National Institutes of Health, the HIV Medicine Association of the Infectious Diseases Society of America, and the Pediatric Infectious Diseases Society. These guidelines are updated regularly to provide current information. The most recent information is available at http://AIDSinfo.nih.gov [2].

Effect of Highly Active Antiretroviral Therapy on Risk and Pattern of Opportunistic Infection

The introduction of protease inhibitors and non-nucleoside reverse transcriptase inhibitors for treatment of HIV infections made possible the use of antiretroviral combinations known as highly active antiretroviral therapy (HAART) [6]. Since the implementation of HAART became widespread, it has changed the natural history of HIV-1 infection in the developed world, the life expectancy of HIV-1-infected adults and children improving sharply [8]. Immune reconstitution engendered by HAART in HIV-positive children has significantly lowered mortality and frequency of bacterial infections and opportunistic infections, such as *Pneumocystic jeroveci* pneumonia (PCP) and disseminated *Mycobacterium avium* complex (DMAC), compared with the pre-HAART era [5]. Descriptions of opportunistic infections in the HAART era among children have been limited.

Advances have been made in laboratory and clinical research related to individual opportunistic infections, and use of HAART has dramatically increased in HIV-infected children, changing the epidemiology and presentation of opportunistic infections among children and adults [7]. In an observational study from pediatric clinical trial sites in the United States, PACTG 219, the incidence of the most common initial OIs in children in the potent HAART era (2000 – 2004) was substantially lower than the incidence in children followed at the same sites during the pre-HAART era (1988 – 1998) [1, 5]. For example, the incidence per 100 child-years for bacterial pneumonia decreased from 11.1 in the pre-HAART era to 2.2 in the HAART era; bacteremia from 3.3 to 0.4; herpes zoster form 2.9 to 1.1; DMAC from 1.8 to 0.14; and PCP from 1.3 to 0.09 [2] .

In another prospective observational study to evaluate the rates and causes of hospitalization and mortality among HIV-infected Thai children after receiving HAART [9] showed that the hospitalization rate decreased from 30.7% during the first 24-week period to 2.0% during weeks 120-144 after initiation of HAART. Causes of hospitalization were pneumonia and other bacterial infections (61.7%), immune reconstitution syndrome (23.4%), noninfectious illness (6.5%), other opportunistic infections (5.6%), and drug-related events (2.8%). The mortality rate decreased from 5.7% in the first 24 weeks to 0%-0.6% in the subsequent 24-week intervals.

In another study from Brazil cohort of 371 children and adolescents reported the significant reduction in the overall rate of opportunistic infections from 18.32 per 100 person year in the pre-HAART period to 2.63 per 100 person year during post-HAART periods [10].

The risk of opportunistic infections decreases in concert with an increase in the CD4 lymphocyte count following initiation of HAART with rates of some OIs, such as mycobacterial diseases and cytomegalovirus disease remaining high for the first 3 months after initiating HAART before declining [11]. Likewise, the Swiss cohort analysis reported that the risk of developing an opportunistic infection for a person receiving potent antiretroviral therapy was highest during the initial months of therapy [12]. In another analysis of PACTG 219C, lack of a sustained response to HAART rather than age at or duration of HAART use is predictive of opportunistic infection risk in children [13].

Immune Reconstitution Syndrome

Immune reconstitution inflammatory syndrome (IRIS) or immune restoration syndrome is a widely recognized phenomenon that can complicate antiretroviral therapy. The case definition for IRS requires two major criteria or one major criteria plus 2 minor criteria. The major criteria are (1) atypical presentation of opportunistic infection responding to HAART e.g. localized disease, exaggerated inflammatory reaction, atypical inflammatory response, or progressive organ dysfunction of pre-existing lesions after definite clinical improvement with pathogen specific therapy before the initiation of HAART; (2) decrease in plasma HIV RNA > 1 log 10 copies per mL. The minor criteria are (1) increase in blood CD4 T cell count after starting ART, (2) increase in an immune response specific to the relevant pathogen and (3) spontaneous resolution of disease without specific antimicrobial therapy with continuation of ART [14]. Pneumonia and other bacterial infections were the principal causes of admission in the pre-HAART era (1994-1995) and continued to be the leading causes until 1999. During 2000-2001, antiretroviral toxicity and immune reconstitution inflammatory syndrome emerged as leading causes of hospitalization, in addition to pneumonia and other bacterial infections [15].

Initiation of HAART in the setting of an acute or latent OI can lead to IRIS, an exaggerated inflammatory reaction that can cause clinical worsening of an existing active, latent, or occult OI, where infectious pathogens that were previously not recognized by the immune system now evoke an immune response and require use of anti-inflammatory drugs [2]. An example is activation of latent or occult TB following initiation of ART (referred to by some experts as "unmasking IRIS"). Alternatively, there can be clinical recrudescence of a successfully treated infection, with a paradoxical, symptomatic relapse despite microbiologic treatment success and sterile cultures (referred to by some experts as "paradoxical IRIS"). In this case, there is reconstitution of antigen-specific T-cell-mediated immunity with activation of the immune system following initiation of HAART against persisting antigens, whether present as dead, intact organisms or debris.

In adolescents and adults, IRIS has most frequently been observed following initiation of HAART in individuals with mycobacterial infections, including MAC and *Mycobacterium tuberculosis*, PCP, cryptococcal infection, CMV, varicella zoster or herpes virus infections, hepatitis B and C infections, toxoplasmosis, and progressive multifocal leukoencephalopathy (PML). In children, reactions have also been described in children who had received *Bacille Calmette-Guerin* (BCG) vaccine and later initiated HAART [16-19].

There is little information about the incidence of IRIS in children, especially from resource-limited countries. The proposed clinical definition of immune reconstitution syndrome is worsening symptoms of inflammation or infection temporally related to initiating HAART, usually occurred in the patient who had virologic and or immunologic response defined as had > 2 $\log_{10}$ decrease in plasma HIV RNA or gain ≥5%. In a study of 153 symptomatic children with CD4<15% at initiation of therapy in Thailand, the incidence of IRIS was 19%, with a median time of onset at 4 weeks after the initiation of HAART. The common causes included mycobacterial organisms, varicella zoster virus, herpes simplex virus, cryptococcus neoformans. Children who developed IRIS had lower baseline CD4 percentage compared to those who did not [20].

No randomized controlled trials have been published evaluating treatment of IRIS, and treatment has been based on severity of disease. For mild cases, observation alone with close clinical and laboratory monitoring may be sufficient. For moderate cases, nonsteroidal anti-inflammatory drugs have been used to ameliorate symptoms. For severe cases, corticosteroids, such as dexamethasone, have been used. However, the optimal dosing and duration of therapy are currently unknown, and inflammation can take weeks to months to subside. During this time HAART should be continued [2].

Specific data to guide recommendations for when to start HAART in the setting of an acute OI in children and the management of HAART when an acute OI occurs in a child already receiving HAART are limited. The decision of when to start HAART in a child with an acute or latent OI needs to be individualized and will vary depending on the degree of immunologic suppression in the child prior to starting HAART. Similarly, in a child already receiving HAART who develops and OI, management will need to take into account the child's clinical, viral, and immune status on HAART and the potential drug-drug interactions between the HAART and the required OI drug regimen [2].

OI Prophylaxis and Discontinue Prophylaxis

Studies in adults and children have demonstrated that HAART reduces the incidence of OIs and improves survival, independent of the use of OI antimicrobial prophylaxis. HAART can lead to the improvement or resolution of certain OIs, particularly ones such as cryptosporidiosis or microsporidiosis infection, where an effective specific treatment is not available. However, potent HAART does not replace the need for OI prophylaxis in children with severe immune suppression [2]. The primary prophylaxis to certain OI should be given (Table 1). Increased understanding of the pathogenesis of HIV and associated opportunistic pathogens has led to effective prophylaxis for many of these infections. Although we are unable to directly estimate the individual effect of antiretroviral therapy and prophylaxis, the combined effect of the 2 are associated with a substancial reduction in the incidence of previously common opportunistic infections [5].

In comparison with recurrent serious bacterial infections, some of the protozoan, fungal, or viral OIs complicating HIV are not curable with available treatments. Sustained, effective HAART, resulting in improved immune status, has been established as the most important factor in control of OIs among both HIV-infected adults and children [21]. For many OIs, following treatment of the initial infectious episode, secondary prophylaxis in the form of suppressive therapy is indicated to prevent recurrent clinical disease from reactivation or reinfection [22]. Before the era of HAART, the OI prophylaxis should be taken for life long. However, after at least 6 months of HAART, the opportunistic infection prophylaxis can be safely discontinued in children with immune reconstitution. In general, primary prophylaxis against *P. jeroveci*, toxoplasmosis, and disseminated *M. avium* complex infection can be safely discontinued in adults and children > 2 years of age following immune reconstitution (CD4 cell percentage of >15%) while receiving stable antiretroviral therapy (Table 1).

Table 1. Criteria to consider opportunistic infection primary prophylaxis and discontinuation of prophylaxis [2]

	Criteria for initiation of primary prophylaxis	Criteria for primary prophylaxis discontinuation	Medication
PCP	HIV-exposed infant under 1 year of age HIV-infected children 1-5 years: CD4 < 500 cells/mm3 or < 15% 6-12 years : CD4 < 200 cells/mm3 or < 15%	Do not discontinue if age < 1 year After > 6 months of HAART and 1-5 years; CD4 > 15% or > 500 cells/mm3 for > 3 consecutive months Age > 6 years, CD4 > 15% or 200 cells/mm3 for > 3 consecutive months	TMP/SMX 150/750 mg/m2 divided into 2 doses given 3 times weekly
Mycobacterium avium complex	Age > 6 years; CD4 < 50 cells/mm^3 Age 2-5 years; CD4 < 75 cells/mm^3 Age 1-2 years; CD4 < 500 cells/mm^3 Age < 1 year; CD4 < 750 cells/mm^3	Do not discontinue in age < 2 years, Age 2-5 years with CD4 > 200 cells/mm^3 for 3 months, Age > 6 years with CD4 > 100 cells/mm3 for 3 months.	Clarithromycin 7.5 mg/kg twice daily or Azithromycin 20 mg/kg weekly
Toxoplasma gondii	Age < 6 year with CD4 < 15% Age > 6 year with CD4 < 100 cells/mm3	Do not discontinue if age < 1 year After > 6 months of HAART and 1-5 years; CD4 > 15% or > 500 cells/mm3 for > 3 consecutive months Age > 6 years, CD4 > 15% or 100-200 cells/mm3 for > 3 consecutive months	TMP-SMX 150/750 mg/m2 daily in 2 divided doses
Tuberculosis	TST ≥ 5 mm OR Close contact with any person with contagious TB.	Not applicable	
Varicella	Substantial exposure to varicella or shingle s with no history of varicella or zoster	Not applicable	Varicella zoster immunoglobuin within 96 hours after exposure
Vaccine preventable diseases	Standard recommendations for immunization, except live attenuated vaccine which should be given to children with CD4 > 15%	Not applicable	

HIV-infected children should be protected from vaccine-preventable diseases. Most vaccines recommended for routine use can be safely administered to HIV-exposed or – infected children. All inactivated vaccines can be administered safely to persons with altered immunocompetence whether the vaccine is a killed whole organism or a recombinant, subunit, toxoid, polysaccharide, or polysaccharide protein-conjugate vaccine. If inactivated vaccines are indicated for persons with altered immunocompetence, the usual doses and schedules are recommended. However, the effectiveness of such vaccinations might be suboptimal [23].

Persons with severe cell-mediated immune deficiency should not receive live attenuated vaccines. However, children with HIV infection are at increased risk for complications of varicella, herpes zoster, and measles compared with immunocompetent children. On the basis of limited safety, immunogenicity, and efficacy data among HIV-infected children, varicella and MMR vaccines can be considered for HIV-infected children who are not severely immunosuppressed (i.e., those with age-specific CD4 cell percentage of >= 15%) [23-25]. The recommended immunization schedules for HIV-exposed and –infected children aged 0 to 6 years and 7 to 18 years were approved by the Advisory Committee on Immunization Practices (ACIP) through October 2007 [2]. These schedules will be updated annually to reflect additional vaccine recommendations that are approved by the ACIP and pertain to HIV-exposed or –infected children.

Treatment of opportunistic infections is an evolving science, and availability of new agents or clinical data on existing agents might change therapeutic options and preferences. As a result, these recommendations will need to be periodically updated [7].

Conclusion

In the era of antiretroviral therapy, declining incidence rates were seen for all OIs. These changes are attributable largely to the widespread use of HAART but also to improvements in care, such as improved identification of at risk infants (through testing of pregnant women), the remarkable decrease in mother-to-child HIV transmission [26], and improved use of OI prophylaxis. It remains to be seen whether these declining trends in OI incidence will be sustained as more children proceed through adolescence and whether a similar pattern of decline in OI incidence will be seen as HAART becomes more available to resource-limited areas.

Despite these current advances due to HAART, some HIV-infected children continue to be at risk of developing opportunistic infections during the first few months of treatment due to low immunity or during late stage due to viral resistance, poor adherence, or inability to tolerate complex treatment regimens. Immune reconstitution inflammatory syndrome, initially described in HIV-infected adults but also seen in HIV-infected children, can complicate treatment of OIs when starting HAART or when trying to optimize a failing regimen in a patient with acute OI. However, in children with immune recovery after HAART can be safely discontinued OI prophylaxis. Thus, the prevention and management of OIs remains critical components of care for HIV-infected children even in an era of HAART.

References

[1] Dankner WM, Lindsey JC, Levin MJ, and the Pediatric AIDS Clinical Trials Group Protocol Teams 051, 128, 138, 144, 152, 179, 190, 220, 240, 245, 254, 300, and 327. Correlates of opportunistic infections in children infected with the human immunodeficiency virus managed before highly active antiretroviral therapy. *Pediatr Infect Dis J* 2001;20(1):40-8.

[2] Recommendations from Centers of Disease Control and Prevention, the National Institutes of Health, the HIV Medicine Association of the Infectious Diseases Society of America, and the Pediatric Infectious Diseases Society. Guidelines for Prevention

and Treatment of Opportunistic Infections among HIV-Exposed and HIV-Infected Children. [cited June 20, 2008]. Available from http://AIDSinfo.nih.gov.

[3] Pancharoen C, Thisyakorn U. Pediatric acquired immunodeficiency syndrome in Asia: Mother-to-child transmission. *Clin Infect Dis J* 2002;34(Suppl 2):S65-S69.

[4] Chansinghakul D, Waidab W, Hiranraj T, Mayurasakorn Y, Hemungkorn S, Thisyakorn U. Slow progression of human immunodeficiency infection in a 14-year-old boy born to an HIV-infected mother. *JPID* 2007;2:105-108.

[5] Gona P, Van Dyke RB, Williams PL, et al. Incidence of opportunistic and other infections in HIV-infected children in the HAART era. *JAMA* 2006;296(3):292-300.

[6] Nesheim SR, Kapogiannis BG, Soe MM, et al. Trends in opportunistic infections in the pre-and post-highly active antiretroviral therapy eras among HIV-infected children in the Perinatal AIDS Collaborative Transmission Study, 1986-2004. *Pediatrics* 2007;120(1):100-9.

[7] Mofenson LM, Oleske J, Serchuck L, Dyke RV, Wilfert C. Treating opportunistic infections among HIV-exposed and infected children: recommendations from CDC, the National Institutes of Health, and the Infectious Diseases Society of America. The most recent information is available at http://aidsinfo.nih.gov. *Clin Infect Dis* 2005;40 (Suppl 1): S1-84.

[8] Chiappini E, Galli L, Tovo PA, et al. Changing patterns of clinical events in perinatally HIV-1-infected children during the era of HAART. *AIDS* 2007;21:1607-15.

[9] Puthanakit T, Aurpibul L, Oberdorfer P, et al. Hospitalization and mortality among HIV-infected children after receiving highly active antiretroviral therapy. *Clin Infect Dis* 2007;44(2):599-604.

[10] Candiani TM, Pinto J. antiretroviral therapy (HAART) on the incidence of opportunistic infections, hospitalizations and mortality among children and adolescents living with HIV/AIDS in Belo Horizonte, Minas Gerais State, Brazil.Cad Saude Publica. 2007;23 Suppl 3:S414,

[11] Finkelstein DM, Williams PL, Molenberghs G, et al. Patterns of opportunistic infections in patients with HIV-infection. *J Acquir Immune Defic Syndr Hum Retrovirol.* 1996;12:38-45.

[12] Ledergerber B, Egger M, Erard V, et al. AIDS-related opportunistic illnesses occurring after initiation of potent antiretroviral therapy: the Swiss HIV Cohort Study. *JAMA* 1999;282:2220-6.

[13] Ylitalo N, Brogly S, Hughes MD, et al. Pediatric AIDS Clinical Trial Group Protocol 219C Team. Risk factors for opportunistic illnesses in children with human immunodeficiency virus in the era of highly active antiretroviral therapy. *Arch Pediatr Adolesc Med* 2006;160:778-87.

[14] French MA, Price P, Stone SF. Immune restoration disease after antiretroviral therapy. AIDS 2004;18:1615-27.

[15] Viani RM, Araneta MRG, Deville JG, Spector SA. Decrease in hospitalization and mortality rates among children with perinatally acquired HIV type 1 infection receiving highly active antiretroviral therapy. *Clin Infect Dis* 2004;39:725-31.

[16] Puthanakit T, Oberdorfer P, Punjaisee S, et al. Immune reconstitution syndrome due to Bacillus Calmette Guerin after initiation of antiretroviral therapy in children with HIV infection. *Clin Infect Dis* 2005;41(7):1049-52.

[17] Puthanakit T, Oberdorfer P, Akarapol N, et al. Immune reconstitution syndrome from nontuberculous mycobacterial infection after initiation of antiretroviral therapy in children with HIV infection. *Pediatr Infect Dis J* 2006;25(7):645-8.

[18] Kroidl A, Huck K, Weinspach S, et al. Immune reconstitution inflammatory syndrome (IRIS) due to Bacillus Calmette Guerin (BCG) in an HIV-positive child. *Scan J Infect Dis* 2006;38(8):716-8.

[19] Alexander A, Rode H. Adverse reactions to the Bacillus Calmette-Guerin vaccine in HIV-positive infants. *J Pediatr Surg* 2007;43(3):549-52.

[20] Puthanakit T, Oberdorfer P, Akarapol N, et al. Immune reconstitution syndrome after highly active antiretroviral therapy in human immunodeficiency virus-infected Thai children. *Pediatr Infect Dis J* 2006;25(1):53-8.

[21] Guidelines for the use of Antiretroviral Agents in Pediatric HIV Infection. October 26, 2006;1-126. http://aidsinfo.nih.gov/ContentFiles/PediatricGuidelines.pdf. Developed by the Working Group on Antiretroviral Therapy and Medical Management of HIV-Infected Children. The most recent information is available at http://aidsinfo.nih.gov.

[22] Kaplan J, Masur H, Holmes K, et al. Guidelines for preventing opportunistic infections among HIV-infected persons--2002. Recommendations of the U.S. Public Health Service and the Infectious Disease Society of America. *MMWR Recomm Rep*;2002.51(RR-8):1-52.

[23] Kroger AT, Atkinson WL, Marcuse EK, et al. General recommendations on immunization: recommendations of the Advisory Committee on Immunization Practices (ACIP). *MMWR Recomm Rep*, 2006.55(RR-15):1-48.

[24] Watson JC, Hadler SC, Dykewicz CA, et al. Measles, mumps, and rubella—vaccine use and strategies for elimination of measles, rubella, and congenital rubella syndrome and control of mumps: recommendations of the Advisory Committee on Immunization Practices (ACIP). *MMWR Recomm Rep*, 1998.47 (RR-8):1-57.

[25] Marin M, Guris D, Chaves SS, et al. Prevention of varicella: recommendations of the Advisory Committee on Immunization Practices (ACIP). *MMWR Recomm Rep*, 2007.56 (RR-4):1-40.

[26] Chansinghakul D, Kulthida S, Chitsanu P, Thaithumyanon P, Limpongsanurak S, Thisyakorn U. Preventation of mother-to-child HIV transmission: MTCT-plus initiative program. In: *Scientific Programme of the 25th International Congress of Pediatrics.* Athens; August 25-30, 2007 [Abstract No. PP0525].

In: AIDS- Related Opportunistic Infections
Editor: Claudia D. Galanda

ISBN: 978-1-60692-144-9

Chapter VI

Tropical Blood Infection in HIV: Evidence for Opportunistic Infection

Viroj Wiwanitkit
Wiwanitkit House, Bangkhae Bangkok, Thailand
Hainan Medical College, China

Abstract

Opportunistic infection is a problem in managing immunodeficiency virus (HIV) infection with severely impaired immune status. A number of infections are documented and more knowledge is required for proper management. At present, HIV infection has a very high prevalence in many tropical developing countries. An important concern is tropical blood infection, which is also common in these countries. A high chance of co-occurrence can be seen. A compelling question remains regarding whether there is any specific implication for the finding of co-occurrence of HIV and tropical blood infections. There is some new recent evidence for opportunistic infection in those co-occurrence cases. In this chapter, the author summarizes tropical blood infection in HIV and further extrapolates to discuss the role of blood infection as opportunistic infection or a strong supporting factor for the vulnerability of HIV-infected patients to opportunistic infection.

Introduction to Blood Infection

The word "blood infection" means a common group of hematological and infectious disorders. Notable examples of blood infections are malaria and babesiosis. Most blood infections are endemic to tropical countries and are significant public health threats in developing countries. However, blood infections can be seen in nontropical countries as well. There is still limited knowledge on this topic, while the wider distribution of the disorder due to globalization can be expected. Most practitioners should realize the need for and be urged to seek information on this topic.

Similar to general disorders in medicine, two main factors contributing to blood infection are inherited and non-inherited factors. Host susceptibility is an important factor. Sometimes blood infections can be seen accompanied with diseases of other systems. Opportunistic infection is a problem in managing human immunodeficiency virus (HIV) infection with severely impaired immune status. A number of infections are documented and more knowledge for proper management is required. At present, HIV infection has a very high prevalence in many tropical developing countries. An important concern is tropical blood infection, also common in these countries. A high chance of co-occurrence can be seen. A compelling questions remains as to whether there is any specific implication for the finding of co-occurrence of HIV and tropical blood infections.

Malaria and HIV

Malaria is a mosquito-borne parasitic infection. It can be said that malaria is a very important tropical mosquito-borne infectious disease. Malaria is caused by protozoan parasites of the genus *Plasmodium*. Four species of *Plasmodium—Plasmodium falciparum, Plasmodium vivax, Plasmodium ovale* and *Plasmodium malariae* can produce the human disease in its various forms. In addition, there are other species that infect animals, such as *Plasmodium gallinaceum*. In humans, malaria is an important and potentially deadly mosquito-borne tropical disease characterized by cyclical bouts of fever with muscle stiffness, shaking and sweating. [1–2]. The interrelation between malaria and HIV infected is summarized below.

1. Epidemiology

HIV seropositive people staying in malaria-endemic areas are at risk for developing severe malaria [3]. Malaria prevention using insecticide-treated bed nets and indoor residual house spraying may be the best available options for these people [3]. Some medical practices for malaria, especially blood transfusion in the treatment of children with anemia from malaria, can be the route for HIV infection, especially in Africa [4–5]. On the other hand, some risk behaviors for HIV infection increase the risk of malaria. Bastos et al. noted that new outbreaks of cases of HIV and malaria were likely to occur among Brazilian injecting-drug users (IDUs), and might conceivably contribute to the development of treatment-resistant strains of malaria in this population [5]. They proposed that health professionals should be alert to this possibility, which could also eventually occur in IDU networks in developed countries [6]. Co-infection might also have facilitated the geographic expansion of malaria in areas where HIV prevalence is high [7]. Abu-Raddad proposed that transient and repeated increases in HIV viral load resulting from recurrent co-infection with malaria might be an important factor in promoting the spread of HIV in sub-Saharan Africa [7]. The coexistence of malaria and HIV infection beyond inhabitants of sub-Saharan Africa, South America and Southeast Asia raises the question whether there is an interaction between these two infections that bring a change in the pathogenesis [8].

2. Pathogenesis

In 2001, Yaffe proposed that chronic latent malaria infection prepared the niche whereby the otherwise feeble HIV coinfection could thrive and cause AIDS [9]. Indeed, acute *P. falciparum* malaria coinfection impacts virus-host dynamics in HIV-1-infected persons at the cellular level, notably showing a reversible induction of HIV-1 replication in CD14 macrophages that is associated with changes in immune activation [10]. Basically, macrophage inflammatory protein-1 alpha (MIP-1 alpha) and MIP-1 beta play an important role in modulating immune responses [11]. Chaisavaneeyakorn et al. reported that MIP-1 beta and MIP-1 alpha levels in PM-positive women were positively associated with parasite density and malaria pigment levels, but HIV infection did not significantly alter these two chemokine levels [11]. However, Chaisavaneeyakorn et al. reported a substantial impairment of interleukin (IL)-12 production in HIV-positive women, implicating this cytokine as a potentially critical regulator of malaria antigen-specific interferon (IFN)-gamma responses in HIV-infected and HIV/placental malaria-coinfected women [12]. In malaria-endemic areas, severe falciparum malaria usually develops after 6 months of age, and most of the CNS manifestations are more common in children over 1 year old [13]. Newton proposed that the coinfection of malaria and HIV-1 might aggravate the neurodevelopmental impairments documented in these children [13].

3. Diagnosis

Diagnosis of co-infection is usually by detection of malaria parasites in red

- blood cells and detection of positive HIV serology. There is no reported on the
- effect of co-infection on the diagnostic test. Slutsker and Marston mentioned
- that malaria wais associated with increases in HIV viral load that, while modest,
- might impact HIV progression or the risk of HIV transmission [14].

4. Treatment

HIV-infected persons are at increased risk for clinical malaria; the risk is greatest when immune suppression is advanced [14]. In tropical countries, immunosupression due to HIV infection has resulted in changes in the clinical presentation of endemic infections [15]. Adults with advanced HIV may be at risk for failure of malaria treatment, especially with sulfa-based therapies [14]. According to the study of Van Geertruyden et al, HIV-1-infected patients with malaria with a CD4 cell count <300 cells/microL have a higher risk of experiencing a recrudescent infection, compared with those with a CD4 cell count >or=300 cells/microL or without HIV-1 infection [16]. Slutsker and Marston mentioned that people with HIV should use cotrimoxazole and insecticide treated mosquito nets [14]. Malaria prevention is particularly important for pregnant women with HIV, although more information is needed about the best combination of strategies for prevention [14]. Increased numbers of doses of intermittent preventive treatment during pregnancy can reduce the risk of placental malaria in women with HIV [14]. Sulfadoxine-pyrimethamine should be prescribed cautiously in women concurrently receiving daily nevirapine and/or zidovudine, and should be avoided in women on daily co-trimoxazole [17]. This should also be applied for the HIV-infected traveler [18].

5. Is Malaria an Oportunistic Infection in HIV?

The question "Is malaria an opportunistic infection in HIV?" is widely discussed. There are many new evidences indicating that malaria becomes more common in the HIV-infected cases with severe impaired CD4 cell count [19–21]. Herrero recently noted that malaria had been implicated in transitory higher viral load and in low CD4 counts, so it could have an influence on higher transmission rates of HIV and perhaps in the course of HIV infection [19]. Wiwanitkit recently proposed a systematic biological approach that both malaria and HIV share a common pathway for immunosuppression [20]. Co-trimoxazole prophylaxis has been shown to be effective in the prevention of some opportunistic infections in HIV-infected patients, but also in prevention of malaria episodes [19]. In addition, antiretroviral protease inhibitors demonstrate antimalarial effects that could have important clinical and therapeutic implications [19]. Patnaik concluded that HIV-infected adults in malaria-endemic areas were at increased risk for malaria [22]. Where possible, additional malaria prevention efforts should be targeted at this population [22].

Filariasis and HIV

Filariasis and dirofilariasis are important tropical mosquito-borne parasitic infections. Filariasis is the name of name for a group of tropical diseases caused by various thread-like parasitic roundworms and their larvae. Filariasis presents with fever, chills, headache, and skin lesions in the early stages and, if untreated, it can progress to include gross enlargement of the limbs and genitalia in a condition called elephantiasis [23]. Several different types of worms are mentioned as causes of filariasis but the common species include the following: *Wucheria bancrofti, Brugia malayi, Onchocerca volvulus, Loa loa, Mansonella streptocerca, Dracunculus medinensis*, *Mansonella pustans*, and *Mansonella ozzardi* [23–24]. However, it should be noted that not all human filariasis diseases are mosquito-borne. The interrelation between filariasis and HIV infected will be summarized

1. Epidemiology

Coinfection between filariasis and HIV can be seen in tropical countries especially for the risk group [25]. According to the study of Bouree et al. on prisoners in France, coinfection between filariasis and HIV could be seen [26]. In Southeast Asia, border bancroftian filariasis caused by *W. bancrofti* nocturnally subperiodic mainly exists in Karens, a hill tribal group residing alongside the Thailand-Myanmar border [27]. Imported bancroftian filariasis caused by *W. bancrofti* nocturnally periodic mainly exists in cross-border Myanmar migrants [27]. A recent report indicated 3.2% of coinfection among these tribes [27].

2.Pathogenesis

Nielsen et al. found that there was a statistically significant positive association between HIV and *W. bancrofti* infection when sex and age were controlled for [28]. This association is likely to reflect underlying mechanisms that need to be clarified to better understand the role of co-infections in HIV pathogenesis [28]. Ballagher et al. proposed that lymphatic filariasis co-infection is associated with increased risk for mother-to-child-transmission of HIV, possibly by a mechanism in which parasite antigens activates lymphocytes in utero [29]. They noted that treatment of helminthic infections during pregnancy might reduce the risk of mother-to-child-transmission of HIV [29]. Multisystem involvement of microfilaria in HIV infection is also reported [30]. However, Brown et al noted that this helminth infection was not associated with more-advanced HIV disease or faster disease progression [31]. They mentioned that antihelminthic therapy might not be beneficial in slowing HIV progression in coinfected adults [31]. Clarification of the possible effect of coinfection on the pathogenesis by further studies is needed.

3. Diagnosis

Diagnosis of co-infection is usually by detection of microfilaria in blood film or antigen detection by immunological method and detection of positive HIV serology. There are some reports on the effect of co-infection on the diagnostic test. Tawill et al found that HIV-infected onchocerciasis patients exhibited significantly impaired antibody responses to *O. volvulus* antigens, and tended to lose their reactivity to these antigens over time due to immune response abnormalities caused by the concomitant HIV infection [32].

4. Treatment

Standard treatment for filariasis is oral antifilarial drugs. The widely used drugs are ivermectin and diethylcarbamazine (DEC). Even in HIV-positive persons with a reduced ratio of CD4+:CD8+ cells and reduced numbers of CD4+ cells, a significant reduction of their microfilaria density was observed after treatment with ivermectin [33]. Thus, in HIV-endemic areas, the usual dose of ivermectin can be administered during mass treatment. Concerning the adverse reaction, ivermectin can be safely used for mass treatment in areas where the prevalences of onchocerciasis and HIV-1 infection are both high [34]. For DEC, effectiveness in those with concomitant HIV is also confirmed [35].

5. Is Filariasis an Opportunistic Infection in HIV?

The question "Is filariasis an opportunistic infection in HIV?" is also widely discussed. However, there are only few evidences on this topic. Of interest, in 2004, Roy et al firstly reported an interesting case with very high microfilarial load (1000/ml) from blood in HIV positive patient, where microfilaria was also demonstrated from the pericardial and pleural fluid and from urine [30]. Therefore, dissseminated filariasis is a suspicious opportunistic infection in HIV.

Babesiosis and HIV

Human babesiosis is caused predominantly by *Babesia microti* and *Babesia divergens*, a protozooan parasites of red blood cells [36]. Both are transmitted by *Ixodes ricinus* ticks, also the primary vector of Lyme disease [36]. Babesia is a tick-transmitted protozoal parasite that can cause malaria-like symptoms and hemolytic anemia [37]. Clinical manifestation varied widely from asymptomatic infection to a serve rapidly fatal disease [36–38]. Asplenic, elderly, and immunocompromised patients are at greatest risk for severe disease; however, babesiosis can be serious in immunologically normal persons [36–38]. The interrelation between babesiosis and HIV infected will be summarized

1. Epidemiology

It is clear that HIV infection is a risk for babesiosis. However, there is no exact epidemiological study to assess the correlation between the epidemiology of babesiosis and HIV.

2. Pathogenesis

As previously mentioned, immunocompromised individuals as a result of immunosuppressive drugs, malignancy, or HIV infection are risk group for babesiosis [39–40]. Babesiosis should be considered in the differential diagnosis of HIV-infected patients with fevers and/or anemia in areas where the infection is endemic [41]. Although the role of HIV coinfection in babesiosis is uncertain, the previously reported cases raise a concern that it may predispose to a more severe clinical course [42]. HIV-infected patients who are severely immunosuppressed, even those without a history of splenectomy, may present with severe manifestations of babesiosis and develop a chronic infection, which may require therapy to prevent relapse of disease [41].

3. Diagnosis

Diagnosis of co-infection is usually by detection of babesia parasites in red blood cells and detection of positive HIV serology. There is no reported on the effect of co-infection on the diagnostic test.

4. Treatment

Babesiosis can be controlled with a maintenance regimen consisting of clindamycin, doxycycline, and high-dose azithromycin, but the infection is usually not eradicated [41]. In severe babesiosis, red blood cell exchange transfusion, combined with appropriate antibiotic therapy, appears to be a rapidly effective therapeutic modality which can induce sustained remissions [42]. Although generally responsive to antibiotic therapy, several cases of severe babesiosis refractory to appropriate antibiotic therapy have been reported to respond promptly and dramatically to red blood cell exchange transfusion [41]. These practices are also applicable for HIV infected cases [41].

5. Is Babesiosis an Opportunistic Infection in HIV?

The question "Is babesiosis is an opportunistic infection in HIV?" is also widely discussed. However, there are only few evidences on this topic. It can be said only that this blood infection is an important cause of fever of unknown origin in HIV-infected patients [41].

Leishmaniasis and HIV

Leishmaniasis is an important tropical vector-borne disease. There are two common forms of leishmaniasis, cutaneous and visceral forms. Leishmanioses are a group of parasitic diseases that affect man and other mammals. They are caused by different species of trypanosomatids of the genus Leishmania [43–44]. Leishmaniasis represents a complex of diseases with a clinical and epidemiological diversity [45]. Leishmaniasis remains a severe public health problem and its burden is increasing [45]. The disease is caused by a parasite belonging to the genus Leishmania [45]. Approximately 350 billion people in 88 different countries are thought to be infected with Leishmania spp. [45]. The distribution of this re-emerging disease, which is found throughout the world (except in Antarctica), is influenced by various factors linked to both human activity and climatic change [44]. Leishmaniasis is still an important public health problem due to not only environmental risk factors such as massive migrations, urbanisation, deforestation, new irrigation schemes, but also to individual risk factors: HIV, malnutrition, genetic, etc. [46]. The interrelation between leishmaniasis and HIV infected will be summarized

1. Epidemiology

Since leishmaniasis is still an important public threat to many tropical developing countries where HIV infection is also endemic, the coinfection can be expected. Mathur et al reported that the reported increase in the prevalence of HIV in the visceral leishmaniasis-endemic and co-infection might assume epidemic proportions in the coming decade if left [47] unchecked. India, Nepal and Ethiopia are the good examples of countries with the problems of the coinfection [47 – 49]. Montalban et al. found that visceral leishmaniasis was an opportunistic disease that should be suspected in HIV-infected patients [50]. They suggested that it should be included in the CDC group IV C-1 and considered as a disease indicative of AIDS [50]. Pintado et al. reported that the clinical presentation of leishmaniasis was similar in both HIV-infected and non HIV-infected patients, but HIV-infected patients had a lower frequency of splenomegaly than HIV-negative individuals [51].

2. Pathogenesis

Protozoan parasites of the genus Leishmania frequently occur as opportunistic pathogens in HIV-1-infected individuals, but the mechanisms underlying protozoan growth in this context are poorly understood [52–53]. In the light of the recent demonstration that L. donovani can up-regulate HIV replication, both in monocytoid and lymphoid cells in vitro and in co-infected individuals, it is clear from the epidemiological data available that Leishmania can probably act as a powerful co-factor in the pathogenesis of HIV infection [54]. In those who are co-infected, complex mechanisms involving cytokine secretion and cellular-signalling events play pivotal roles in the Leishmania-mediated activation and pathogenesis of HIV [54]. HIV infection appears to have a more profound impact on the development of visceral leishmaniasis than on the evolution of the purely cutaneous disease [55]. Co-infection of HIV and visceral leishmaniasis and their interdependence has been addressed [56]. Enhanced expression of the human immunodeficiency virus (HIV) co-receptor CXCR4 renders T-lymphocytes more susceptible for infection with HIV [52].

Barreto-de-Souza et al suggested that Tat generated a milieu permissive to Leishmania growth in individuals infected with HIV-1 [53]. Following the dissemination of the parasites, the HIV-positive cases may develop unusual, multi-organ pathology [57]. Almost all the cases of co-infection are very prone to visceral leishmaniasis relapses, even after carefully managed antileishmanial treatment [57]. The opportunistic infections that are often seen in HIV-positives frequently develop during visceral leishmaniasis episodes, the signs and symptoms of the leishmaniasis then confusingly overlapping with those of the other infections [57].

3. Diagnosis

Diagnosis of visceral leishmaniasis relies on demonstration of the parasite in bone marrow specimens or in the spleen [58]. The parasite demonstration and isolation rates are rather poor from cutaneous and mucocutaneous lesions due to low parasite load and high rate of culture contamination [59]. Serologic testing is useful with the indirect fluorescent antibody test (IFAT), [60]. Pintado et al. reported that the sensitivity of serologic studies for Leishmania was significantly lower in HIV-infected than in non-HIV-infected patients, but the diagnostic yield of bone marrow aspirate and bone marrow culture (62.9% versus 66.6%) was similar in both groups [51]. Present data stress the utility of the follow-up by Western blotting for an early diagnosis of visceral leishmaniasis, and therefore an early treatment, for HIV-positive patients living in endemic areas [61]. Kubar et al. suggested that in a latent leishmania infection supplementary control mechanism might operate in addition to the T-cell-mediated response, and provide a further example of non-appearance of an opportunistic infection despite a severe reduction in CD4+ T cells [61].

Recently several recombinant proteins have been developed to accomplish accurate diagnosis. Recombinant kinesin protein of 39 kDa called rK 39 is the most promising of these molecules. The antigen used in various test formats has been proved highly sensitive and specific for visceral leishmaniasis [59]. It is useful in the diagnosis of HIV-Leishmania co-infection and as a prognostic marker [59].

4. Treatment

Although leishmaniasis could contribute to death in a significant number of HIV-infected patients, it was the main cause of death in only a few of them. The CD4+ lymphocyte count and the use of highly active antiretroviral therapy and secondary prophylaxis for leishmaniasis were the most significant prognostic factors for survival in AIDS patients [51]. Combination of two most potent leishmanicidal drugs amphotericin B and miltefosine which are not dependent on host immune system, may shorten the course of therapy besides encountering unresponsiveness [62]. A combination therapy should be preferred when treating kala-azar associated with HIV/AIDS. In a comparative trial, amphotericin B lipid complex was found to be not only as effective as a pentavalent antimonial but also better tolerated [63 - 64]. Although the data available on secondary prophylaxis are limited and often inconclusive, it appears that regular treatment with a pentavalent antimonial drug, liposomal amphothericin B or amphotericin B lipid complex can reduce the incidence of leishmanial relapses in HIV-positive patients with leishmaniasis [64]. A different immune response was noticed in patients with co-infection of HIV and leishmania [63]. Antileishmanial drug treatment led to improvement in immunological response in co-infected patients [63]. Pintado et al found that the response rate was significantly lower in HIV-infected than in non-HIV-infected individuals after initial treatment [51]. The development of new regimens, use of new oral drugs (such as miltefosine) and the development of new antileishmanial drugs could all improve the treatment of HIV-related visceral leishmaniasis in the future [64].

5. Is Leismaniasis an Opportunistic Infection in HIV ?

The question "Is leismaniasis an opportunistic infection in HIV?" is also widely discussed. There are several studies published about Leishmania/HIV co-infection, however some particularities of its epidemiology, pathogenesis and especially of its treatment and prophylaxis remain unclear and undefined [65]. Marques et al. suggested that visceral leishmaniasis behaved as an opportunistic infection in HIV-infected patients and should be considered as an AIDS-defining disease [65].

Trypanosomiasis and HIV

Trypanosomiasis is an important vector borne blood infection. The pathogenic organisms causing trypanosomiasis is the parasite in the genus Trypanosoma. In the peripheral blood smear, it is usually characterized by an undulating membrane. There are three main medically important species: *Trypanosoam brucei gambiense*, *T. brucei rhodesiense* and *T. cruzi*. There are three main types of trypanosomiasis: African sleeping sickness caused by *Trypanosoam gambiense*, East African sleeping sickness caused by *T. rhodesiense* and Chagas disease caused by *T. cruzi*. Africa is the main endemic area for trypanosomiasis [66–67]. Research on the disease suggests that the development of a vaccine is still far away; even existing drugs are becoming ineffective on account of the emergence of drug-resistant trypanosomes [67–68]. The interrelation between trypanosomiasis and HIV infected will be summarized

1. Epidemiology

Similar to leishmaniasis, trypanosomiasis is still an important public threat to many tropical developing countries where HIV infection is also endemic, the coinfection can be expected. Pepin et al suggest that HIV-1 infection was not having a significant impact on the incidence of *T. brucei* gambiense sleeping sickness e, but the possibility that incident cases of trypanosomiasis concurrently infected with HIV-1 may be at higher risk of treatment failure warranted further investigation [69].

2. Pathogenesis

Cerebral Chagas' disease can be considered another potential opportunistic infection in AIDS resulting from the reactivation of a dormant *T. cruzi* infection acquired years earlier [70]. Although immunosuppression is observed, with CD4 T lymphocytes below 200/micron^3, these HIV-infected patients do not display reactivation of *T. cruzi* infection and that a balance favorable to Th2 is associated with the presence of parasitemia [71]. Recent evidence from patients with HIV/AIDS indicates that CD28-cell populations are more likely to undergo apoptosis, and increased apoptosis has been observed in experimental Chagas disease [72].

3. Diagnosis

Demonstration of the causal agent is the diagnostic procedure in trypanosomasis. The peripheral blood smear examination becomes a useful simple test for diagnosis of trypanosomiasis. A serological test is also useful for diagnosis. Indirect immunofluorescence test in trypanosomiasis is usually positive at 1:20 and higher dilutions, even in the presence of concomitant infection with HIV [73]. Although there has been an improvement in the diagnosis of chronic trypanosomiasis, the low sensitivity of indirect parasitological tests is a drawback to its application in diagnosis and post-therapeutic control [74]. Polymerase chain reaction (PCR) has limited use in routine diagnosis due to the need for specific laboratory facilities, common DNA cross-contamination, and high costs [74].

4. Treatment

In general, specific antitrypanosomal treatment with benznidazole is effective in reducing the level of parasitemia and improving the clinical condition. This also applies to HIV-infected cases [75]. Such patients, when treated, appear to recover from trypanosomiasis but later succumb to full-blown AIDS [76]. It is recommended that CD4+ T cell numbers and CD4/CD8 T cell ratios be assessed to investigate response to treatment in HIV-positive trypanosomiasis patients [76]. Benznidazole is also useful for treatment of cerebral trypanosomiasis in HIV-infected patients [77–78].

5. Is Trypanosomiasis an Opportunistic Infection in HIV ?

The question "Is trypanosomiasis an opportunistic infection in HIV?" is also widely discussed. Chagasic meningitis is a severe form of trypanosomiasis that can be seen in HIV-infected cases [79–80]. Along with leishmaniasis, trypanosomiasis is presented as an opportunistic infection in HIV [81].

Conclusion

Blood infection is defined as a common group of hematological and infectious disorders. A notable example is the occurrence of blood infection in the patient with HIV infection. The effects of blood infections on the epidemiology, pathogenesis, diagnosis and treatment of HIV infection can be expected. On the other hand, the effect of HIV infection on the epidemiology, pathogenesis, diagnosis and treatment of those blood infections can also be expected. In this chapter, the interrelation between blood infection and HIV infection was summarized and discussed. An important question remains regarding whether there is any specific implication for the finding of co-occurrence of HIV and tropical blood infections. There is some new recent evidence for opportunistic infection in those co-occurrence cases. In this chapter, the author summarized the tropical blood infection in HIV and further extrapolated to discuss the role of blood infection as opportunistic infection or a strong supporting factor for HIV-infected patients to be vulnerable to opportunistic infection.

References

[1] Chareonviriyaphap T, Bangs MJ, Ratanatham S. Status of malaria in Thailand. *Southeast Asian J Trop Med Public Health*. 2000; 31: 225-37.

[2] Phillips RS. Current status of malaria and potential for control. *Clin Microbiol*. 2001; 14: 208-26.

[3] Chirenda J, Murugasampillay S. Malaria and HIV co-infection: available evidence, gaps and possible interventions. *Cent Afr J Med*. 2003;49:66-71.

[4] Piot P, Carael M. Epidemiological and sociological aspects of HIV-infection in developing countries. *Br Med Bull*. 1988;44:68-88.

[5] Fleming AF. HIV and blood transfusion in sub-Saharan Africa. *Transfus Sci*. 1997;18:167-79.

[6] Bastos FI, Barcellos C, Lowndes CM, Friedman SR. Co-infection with malaria and HIV in injecting drug users in Brazil: a new challenge to public health? *Addiction*. 1999; 94: 1165-74.

[7] Abu-Raddad LJ, Patnaik P, Kublin JG. Dual infection with HIV and malaria fuels the spread of both diseases in sub-Saharan Africa. *Science*. 2006;314:1603-6.

[8] Siwak E, Kowalczuk-Kot A, Pogorzelska J. Malaria and HIV co-infection. *Wiad Parazytol*. 2006;52:9-11.

[9] Yaffe I. AIDS possibly caused by HIV and latent malaria coinfection. *Med Hypotheses*. 2001;57:419-22.

[10] Pisell TL, Hoffman IF, Jere CS, Ballard SB, Molyneux ME, Butera ST, Lawn SD. Immune activation and induction of HIV-1 replication within CD14 macrophages during acute Plasmodium falciparum malaria coinfection. *AIDS*. 2002;16:1503-9.

[11] Chaisavaneeyakorn S, Moore JM, Mirel L, Othoro C, Otieno J, Chaiyaroj SC, Shi YP, Nahlen BL, Lal AA, Udhayakumar V. Levels of macrophage inflammatory protein 1 alpha (MIP-1 alpha) and MIP-1 beta in intervillous blood plasma samples from women with placental malaria and human immunodeficiency virus infection. *Clin Diagn Lab Immunol*. 2003;10:631-6.

[12] Chaisavaneeyakorn S, Moore JM, Otieno J, Chaiyaroj SC, Perkins DJ, Shi YP, Nahlen BL, Lal AA, Udhayakumar V. Immunity to placental malaria. III. Impairment of interleukin(IL)-12, not IL-18, and interferon-inducible protein-10 responses in the placental intervillous blood of human immunodeficiency virus/malaria-coinfected women. *J Infect Dis*. 2002;185:127-31.

[13] Newton CR. Interaction between Plasmodium falciparum and human immunodeficiency virus type 1 on the central nervous system of African children. *J Neurovirol*. 2005;11 Suppl 3:45-51.

[14] Slutsker L, Marston BJ. HIV and malaria: interactions and implications. *Curr Opin Infect Dis*. 2007;20:3-10.

[15] Suri V, Bhalla A, Sharma N, Jain S, Varma S. HIV immunosupression and malaria: is there a correlation? *Indian J Med Sci*. 2006;60:376-9.

[16] McCarthy AE, Mileno MD. Prevention and treatment of travel-related infections in compromised hosts. *Curr Opin Infect Dis*. 2006;19:450-5.

[17] Brentlinger PE, Behrens CB, Micek MA. Challenges in the concurrent management of malaria and HIV in pregnancy in sub-Saharan Africa. *Lancet Infect Dis*. 2006;6:100-11.
[18] Van Geertruyden JP, Mulenga M, Mwananyanda L, Chalwe V, Moerman F, Chilengi R, Kasongo W, Van Overmeir C, Dujardin JC, Colebunders R, Kestens L, D'Alessandro U. HIV-1 immune suppression and antimalarial treatment outcome in Zambian adults with uncomplicated malaria. *J Infect Dis*. 2006;194:917-25.
[19] Herrero MD, Rivas P, Rallón NI, Ramírez-Olivencia G, Puente S. HIV and malaria. *AIDS Rev*. 2007 Apr-Jun;9(2):88-98.
[20] Wiwanitkit V. Co-infection between syphilis and malaria: immune deterioration on CD4+ count. *Irn J Med Hypotheses Ideas* 2008, 2:1.
[21] French N, Nakiyingi J, Lugada E, Watera C, Whitworth JA, Gilks CF._Increasing rates of malarial fever with deteriorating immune status in HIV-1-infected Ugandan adults. *AIDS*. 2001 May 4;15(7):899-906.
[22] Patnaik P, Jere CS, Miller WC, Hoffman IF, Wirima J, Pendame R, Meshnick SR, Taylor TE, Molyneux ME, Kublin JG. Effects of HIV-1 serostatus, HIV-1 RNA concentration, and CD4 cell count on the incidence of malaria infection in a cohort of adults in rural Malawi. *J Infect Dis*. 2005 Sep 15;192(6):984-91.
[23] Filariasis. Available at http://www.chclibrary.org/micromed/00048410.html
[24] Ottesen EA. Lymphatic filariasis: Treatment, control and elimination. *Adv Parasitol*. 2006;61:395-441.
[25] HTLV1 and coinfections. Med Trop (Mars). 1991;51:399-406.
[26] Bouree P, Espinoza P, Coco Cianci O, Loue P. Prevalence of parasitic diseases and HBV and HIV viruses among black Africans in prison. (Study of 116 subjects). *Bull Soc Pathol Exot Filiales*. 1988;81:173-82.
[27] Bhumiratana A, Koyadun S, Srisuphanunt M, Satitvipawee P, Limpairojn N, Gaewchaiyo G. Border and imported bancroftian filariases: baseline seroprevalence in sentinel populations exposed to infections with Wuchereria bancrofti and concomitant HIV at the start of diethylcarbamazine mass treatment in Thailand. *Southeast Asian J Trop Med Public Health*. 2005;36:390-407.
[28] Nielsen NO, Simonsen PE, Magnussen P, Magesa S, Friis H. Cross-sectional relationship between HIV, lymphatic filariasis and other parasitic infections in adults in coastal northeastern Tanzania. *Trans R Soc Trop Med Hyg*. 2006;100:543-50.
[29] Gallagher M, Malhotra I, Mungai PL, Wamachi AN, Kioko JM, Ouma JH, Muchiri E, King CL. The effects of maternal helminth and malaria infections on mother-to-child HIV transmission. *AIDS*. 2005;19:1849-55.
[30] Roy I, Mukhopadhyay C, Ayyagari A. Multisystem involvement of microfilaria in a HIV positive patient. *Nepal Med Coll J*. 2004;6:64-6.
[31] Brown M, Kizza M, Watera C, Quigley MA, Rowland S, Hughes P, Whitworth JA, Elliott AM. Helminth infection is not associated with faster progression of HIV disease in coinfected adults in Uganda. *J Infect Dis*. 2004;190:1869-79.
[32] Tawill SA, Gallin M, Erttmann KD, Kipp W, Bamuhiiga J, Buttner DW. Impaired antibody responses and loss of reactivity to Onchocerca volvulus antigens by HIV-seropositive onchocerciasis patients. *Trans R Soc Trop Med Hyg*. 1996;90:85-9.

[33] Fischer P, Kipp W, Kabwa P, Buttner DW. Onchocerciasis and human immunodeficiency virus in western Uganda: prevalences and treatment with ivermectin. *Am J Trop Med Hyg*. 1995;53:171-8.
[34] Kipp W, Bamhuhiiga J, Rubaale T, Kabagambe G. Adverse reactions to the ivermectin treatment of onchocerciasis patients: does infection with the human immunodeficiency virus play a role? *Ann Trop Med Parasitol*. 2005;99:395-402.
[35] Bhumiratana A, Koyadun S, Srisuphanunt M, Satitvipawee P, Limpairojn N, Gaewchaiyo G. Border and imported bancroftian filariases: baseline seroprevalence in sentinel populations exposed to infections with Wuchereria bancrofti and concomitant HIV at the start of diethylcarbamazine mass treatment in Thailand. *Southeast Asian J Trop Med Public Health*. 2005;36:390-407
[36] Cichocka A, Skotarczak B. Babesosis--difficulty of diagnosis. *Wiad Parazytol*. 2001;47:527-33.
[37] Babesia research. Available on www.vetmed.ucdavis.edu/VBDP/BABESIA.HTM
[38] Gray JS. Babesia sp.: emerging intracellular parasites in Europe. *Pol J Microbiol*. 2004;53 Suppl:55-60.
[39] Krause PJ. Babesiosis. Med Clin North Am. 2002;86:361-73.
[40] Gorenflot A, Moubri K, Precigout E, Carcy B, Schetters TP. Human babesiosis. *Ann Trop Med Parasitol*. 1998;92:489-501.
[41] Falagas ME, Klempner MS. Babesiosis in patients with AIDS: a chronic infection presenting as fever of unknown origin. *Clin Infect Dis*. 1996;22:809-12.
[42] Machtinger L, Telford SR 3rd, Inducil C, Klapper E, Pepkowitz SH, Goldfinger D. Treatment of babesiosis by red blood cell exchange in an HIV-positive, splenectomized patient. *J Clin Apher*. 1993;8:78-81.
[43] Murray HW, Berman JD, Davies CR, Saravia NG. Advances in leishmaniasis. *Lancet* 2005;366:1561-77.
[44] Gallego M. Emerging parasitic zoonoses: leishmaniosisRev Sci Tech. 2004;23:661-76.
[45] Yurdakul P. Immunopathogenesis of Leishmania infections. *Mikrobiyol Bul*. 2005;39:363-81.
[46] Woodruff AW. Recent work concerning anemia in the tropics. *Semin Hematol*. 1982;19:141-7.
[47] Mathur P, Samantaray JC, Vajpayee M, Samanta P. Visceral leishmaniasis/human immunodeficiency virus co-infection in India: the focus of two epidemics. *J Med Microbiol*. 2006;55:919-22.
[48] Gurubacharya RL, Gurubacharya SM, Gurubacharya DL, Quinkel J, Gurubacharya VL. Prevalence of visceral leishmania & HIV co-infection in Nepal. *Indian J Med Res*. 2006;123:473-5.
[49] Anema A, Ritmeijer K. Treating HIV/AIDS and leishmaniasis coinfection in Ethiopia. *CMAJ*. 2005;172:1434-5.
[50] Montalban C, Calleja JL, Erice A, Laguna F, Clotet B, Podzamczer D, Cobo J, Mallolas J, Yebra M, Gallego A. Visceral leishmaniasis in patients infected with human immunodeficiency virus. Co-operative Group for the Study of Leishmaniasis in AIDS. *J Infect*. 1990;21:261-70.

[51] Pintado V, Martin-Rabadan P, Rivera ML, Moreno S, Bouza E. Visceral leishmaniasis in human immunodeficiency virus (HIV)-infected and non-HIV-infected patients. A comparative study. *Medicine* (Baltimore). 2001;80:54-73.

[52] Hailu A, Pater JM, Kager PA, van der Poll T. Increased expression of HIV co-receptor CXCR4 on CD4+ T-cells in patients with active visceral leishmaniasis. *Scand J Infect Dis*. 2004;36:56-8.

[53] Barreto-de-Souza V, Pacheco GJ, Silva AR, Castro-Faria-Neto HC, Bozza PT, Saraiva EM, Bou-Habib DC. Increased Leishmania replication in HIV-1-infected macrophages is mediated by tat protein through cyclooxygenase-2 expression and prostaglandin E2 synthesis. *J Infect Dis*. 2006;194:846-54.

[54] Olivier M, Badaro R, Medrano FJ, Moreno J. The pathogenesis of Leishmania/HIV co-infection: cellular and immunological mechanisms. *Ann Trop Med Parasitol*. 2003;97 Suppl 1:79-98

[55] Deniau M, Canavate C, Faraut-Gambarelli F, Marty P. The biological diagnosis of leishmaniasis in HIV-infected patients. *Ann Trop Med Parasitol*. 2003;97 Suppl 1:115-33.

[56] Salotra P, Singh R. Immune responses in kala-azar. Indian J Med Res. 2006;123:245-66.

[57] Russo R, Laguna F, Lopez-Velez R, Medrano FJ, Rosenthal E, Cacopardo B, Nigro L.Visceral leishmaniasis in those infected with HIV: clinical aspects and other opportunistic infections. *Ann Trop Med Parasitol*. 2003;97 Suppl 1:99-105

[58] Lagardere B, Chevallier B, Cheriet R. Kala-azar. Ann Pediatr (Paris). 1992;39:15964.

[59] Singh S, Sivakumar R. Recent advances in the diagnosis of leishmaniasis. *J Postgrad Med*. 2003;49:55-60.

[60] Leishmaniasis. Available online at http://www.emedicine.com/emerg/topic296.htm

[61] Kubar J, Marty P, Lelievre A, Quaranta JF, Staccini P, Caroli-Bosc C, Le Fichoux Y. Visceral leishmaniosis in HIV-positive patients: primary infection, reactivation and latent infection. Impact of the CD4+ T-lymphocyte counts. *AIDS*. 1998;12:2147-53.

[62] Jha TK. Drug unresponsiveness & combination therapy for kala-azar. *Indian J Med Res*. 2006;123:389-98.

[63] Sinha PK, Bimal S, Singh SK, Pandey K, Gangopadhyay DN, Bhattacharya SK. Pre- & post-treatment evaluation of immunological features in Indian visceral leishmaniasis (VL) patients with HIV co-infection. *Indian J Med Res*. 2006;123:197-202.

[64] Laguna F. Treatment of leishmaniasis in HIV-positive patients. *Ann Trop Med Parasitol*. 2003 Oct;97 Suppl 1:135-42.

[65] Marques N, Cabral S, Sá R, Coelho F, Oliveira J, Saraiva da Cunha JG, Meliço Silvestre_A. Visceral leishmaniasis and HIV infection in the HAART era. *Acta Med Port*. 2007 Jul-Aug;20(4):291-8.

[66] Nok AJ. Effective measures for controlling trypanosomiasis. *Expert Opin Pharmacother*. 2005;6:2645-53.

[67] African sleeping sickness. Available online at http://www.emedicine.com/med/topic2140.htm

[68] Trypanosoma cruzi. Available online at http://www.dbbm.fiocruz.br/tropical/chagas/chapter3.html

[69] Pepin J, Ethier L, Kazadi C, Milord F, Ryder R. The impact of human immunodeficiency virus infection on the epidemiology and treatment of Trypanosoma brucei gambiense sleeping sickness in Nioki, Zaire. *Am J Trop Med Hyg*. 1992;47:133-40.

[70] Pacheco RS, Ferreira MS, Machado MI, Brito CM, Pires MQ, Da-Cruz AM, Coutinho SG. Chagas' disease and HIV co-infection: genotypic characterization of the Trypanosoma cruzi strain. *Mem Inst Oswaldo Cruz*. 1998;93:165-9.

[71] Rodrigues DB, Correia D, Marra MD, Giraldo LE, Lages-Silva E, Silva-Vergara ML, Barata CH, Rodrigues Junior V. Cytokine serum levels in patients infected by human immunodeficiency virus with and without Trypanosoma cruzi coinfection. *Rev Soc Bras Med Trop*. 2005;38:483-7.

[72] Dutra WO, Martins-Filho OA, Cancado JR, Pinto-Dias JC, Brener Z, Gazzinelli G, Carvalho JF, Colley DG. Chagasic patients lack CD28 expression on many of their circulating T lymphocytes. *Scand J Immunol*. 1996;43:88-93.

[73] Portela-Lindoso AA, Shikanai-Yasuda MA. Chronic Chagas' disease: from xenodiagnosis and hemoculture to polymerase chain reaction. *Rev Saude Publica*. 2003; 37:107-15.

[74] Amato Neto V, De Marchi CR, Rossitto ST, Nascimento MS. Evaluation of the sensitivity of the indirect immunofluorescence test at the 1:20 dilution in the diagnosis of Chagas disease. *Rev Soc Bras Med Trop*. 2002;35:195-6.

[75] Sartori AM, Shikanai-Yasuda MA, Amato Neto V, Lopes MH. Follow-up of 18 patients with human immunodeficiency virus infection and chronic Chagas' disease, with reactivation of Chagas' disease causing cardiac disease in three patients. *Clin Infect Dis*. 1998;26:177-9.

[76] Matete GO, Kajejo OA. Human African trypanosomiasis and human immunodeficiency virus co-infection in Western Kenya. *East Afr Med J*. 2005;82:20-3.

[77] Antunes AC, Cecchini FM, Bolli FB, Oliveira PP, Reboucas RG, Monte TL, Fricke D. Cerebral trypanosomiasis and AIDS. *Arq Neuropsiquiatr*. 2002;60:730-3.

[78] Galhardo MC, Martins IA, Hasslocher-Moreno A, Xavier SS, Coelho JM, Junqueira AC, dos Santos RR. Reactivation of Trypanosoma cruzi infection in patients with acquired immunodeficiency syndrome. *Rev Soc Bras Med Trop*. 1999;32:291-4.

[79] Walker M, Kublin JG, Zunt JR. Parasitic central nervous system infections in immunocompromised hosts: malaria, microsporidiosis, leishmaniasis, and African trypanosomiasis. *Clin Infect Dis*. 2006 Jan 1;42(1):115-25.

[80] Lazo J, Meneses AC, Rocha A, Ferreira MS, Marquez JO, Chapadeiro E, Lopes ER. Chagasic meningoencephalitis in the immunodeficient. *Arq Neuropsiquiatr*. 1998 Mar;56(1):93-7.

[81] Dedet JP, Pratlong F. Chagas' disease and HIV co-infection: genotypic characterization of the Trypanosoma cruzi strain. *Mem Inst Oswaldo Cruz*. 1998 Mar-Apr;93(2):165-9.

In: AIDS- Related Opportunistic Infections
Editor: Claudia D. Galanda
ISBN: 978-1-60692-144-9

Chapter VII

Opportunistic Infection in HIV Infection: A Summary of Reports from Thailand

Viroj Wiwanitkit
Wiwanitkit House, Bangkhae Bangkok, Thailand
Hainan Medical College, China

Abstract

Opportunistic infection is an important complication in the course of human immunodeficiency virus (HIV) infection. Opportunistic infection is common for the HIV-infected cases with impaired immune status. A number of infections have been documented and are the focus in HIV medicine. Although the pattern of opportunistic infections in different parts of the world share some common characteristics, the difference among various regions is still an area of interest at present. In this work, the author summarized reports from Thailand on oppportunistic infection in HIV infection. The four main groups of opportunistic infections are the focus of this chapter: respiratory tract infections, neurological infections, skin infections and gastrointestinal infections. It can be shown that opportunistic infection is important in coping with HIV-infected cases in Thailand. In addition, practitioners who deal with patients from Thailand and nearby tropical countries should be aware of the significance of tropical infections as opportunistic infections in HIV-infected cases in Thailand.

Prevalence of Human Immunodeficiency Virus Infection in Thailand

Thailand is a country in Southeast Asia currently facing a high prevalence of human immunodeficiency virus (HIV) infection. Millions of people are believed to be afflicted with

HIV infection in Thailand. There are some reports on the prevalence of HIV infection in Thailand that should be mentioned.

1. HIV Prevalence in the Pregnant Group

There are several reports indicating a high prevalence of HIV infection among the pregnant in Thailand. The first AIDS case was reported in Thailand in 1984 and the first HIV positive pregnant woman delivered her baby at Bamrasnaradura hospital, Nonthaburi province, in October 1988. After this situation, the department of obstetrics and gynecology adopted a policy requiring blood sampling for HIV antibody in all antenatal (ANC) cases since March 1989 [1]. The important reports are shown in Table 1.

Table 1. Reports on the prevalence of HIV infection among pregnant women in Thailand

Authors	Details
Visikijakan [1]	The prevalence of HIV in pregnant women in Bamrasnaradura Hospital prenatal clinic in the early period during which HIV infection emerged in Thailand was reported [1]. This retrospective study showed that 8,772 ANC pregnant women were HIV positive in 23 cases (0.26 %) [1]. The prevalence by year is 0, 0.13, 0.40, and 0.7 % from 1989 to 1992, respectively [1]. Visikijakan proposed that private ANC treatment and counseling should be provided to all HIV-positive pregnant women [1].
Menakanit and Yossing [2]	The objective was to study the prevalence rate of HIV infection in 1,000 pregnant women in Udornthani Hospital from 1–30 November, 1991 [2]. The results were as follows: HIV infection rate in pregnant women was 1% [2]. Most of the patients were under the age of 25, primigravida, low education and worked as employees [2]. The risk factors were mostly sexual promiscuity (50 %) [2]. Outcome of pregnancy: 80% delivered a well baby without congenital abnormality [2]. It was proposed that HIV infection in the pregnant had become an intensified problem [2]. Menakanit and Yossing proposed that prevention and control of HIV infection should be urgently strengthened for reduction of HIV infection in pregnant women and newborns [2].
Sutheeravute [3]	In this work, 2,989 pregnant women who attended at antenatal care unit in Samutsakhon Hospital during January 1991 to March 1992 were studied for hepatitis B, syphilis and HIV [3]. According to the study, 19 cases (0.64 %) were positive for anti-HIV antibodies [3]. Based on the high prevalence found in this study, it is suggested that all of three of these diseases be screened in pregnant women in Samutsakhon Hospital [3].
Jirapinyo et al. [4]	Anti-HIV screening has routinely been done at the antenatal clinic in Ramathibodi Hospital, Bangkok since January 1990 [4]. The prevalence of positive anti-HIV during the first and second half of 1990 and the first half of 1991 are 0.056, 0.2, 0.24 % ,respectively [4]. This study showed that the prevalence of positive anti-HIV was dramatically increasing in that period [4].
Chaiworapongsa and Leelapattana [5]	To assess AIDS infection among pregnant women in Pramongkutklao Hospital and to obtain more data for futher epidemiologic study, a descriptive study was done in 1,500 pregnant women who first attended antenatal clinic from 1st June to 20th October 1992 by having routine laboratory tests including HIV-antibody and self-completing questionnaires [5]. From this study, 66.7 % of seropositive cases could not be identified any risks, therefore, counseling and testing for HIV infection should be offered routinely to all pregnant women [5].

Table 1. (Continued)

Authors	Details
Kuanhin [6]	The study aimed to determine the prevalence and risk markers of HIV infection among pregnant women who attended ANC in a southern province of Thailand [6]. The descriptive study was conducted in five district-community hospitals. Demographic information and HIV status of all pregnant women who attended ANC clinics, during the one year period between June 1995 to May 1996, were retrieved and analyzed [6]. The overall prevalence of HIV infection was 1.27 % (41/3220) [6]. According to this work, there was no statistical assosiation found between HIV infection and other demographic data neither by age, religion, education, occupation, history of abortion nor syphilis infection [6].
Piyapromdee [7]	The aim of this work is to determine the prevalence rate of anemia, syphilitic, hepatitis B virus and HIV infections in pregnant women attending ANC unit at Maharat Nakhon Ratchasima Regional Hospital and Medical Center by retrospective study [7]. In this work, 14,963 pregnant women attending ANC unit for the first time between January 1, 1992 and December 31, 1993 were studied [7]. The prevalence of Hiv infection is equal to 0.46 % [7].

2. HIV Prevalence in the Pediatric Group

As seen in Table 1, the prevalence of HIV infection was somewhat high in the early history of HIV infection in Thailand. Therefore, the next affected group that should be mentioned is the pediatric group. However, there are few reports on HIV prevalence among this population.

3. HIV Prevalence in the Blood Donor Group

Because HIV infection is transmitted by blood, it is a major concern for transfusion medicine. Basically, a blood donor is classified as a representation of healthy adult subjects. The occult HIV infection among this population is considered serious, and screening is recommended. There are some reports on the prevalence of HIV among Thai blood donors. Details of important studies are presented in Table 2.

Opportunistic Infection among HIV-Infected Cases in Thailand

Basically, opportunistic infection is an important complication in the course of HIV infection. The opportunistic infection is common for the HIV-infected cases with impaired immune status. A number of infections are documented and have become the focus in HIV medicine. Although the pattern of opportunistic infections in different parts of the world share some common characteristics, the difference among regions is still an area of interest at present. In Thailand, a country with a high prevalence of HIV infection, there are many reports on opportunistic infection in cases of HIV. The author has summarized the reports from Thailand on oppportunistic infection in HIV infection. The four main groups of opportunistic infections are respiratory tract infections, neurological infections, skin infections and gastrointestinal infections.

Table 2. Teports on prevalence of HIV infection among blood donors in Thailand

Authors	Details
Wattanachote [8]	The prevalence of HIV infection among blood donors studied at Rajavithi Hospital whose blood test for anti HIV done since October 1987 was found out that, in the beginning of the test, October 1987 to December 1988, none of anti HIV was positive among 3,143 blood donors [8]. And in the next year, January to December 1990, anti HIV positive was 30 cases among 3,984 cases of blood donors, the prevalence rate was 0.75 per cent, all were also male [8]. A dramatical increasing can be seen in this work [8].
Archavarungson [9]	The aim of this work is to study the prevalence and trends of copositive of infectious markers in donated blood of Vajira Hospital [9]. A total of 32,147 serum samples were obtained from blood donors during January 1994 to December 1998 at The Blood Bank of Vajira Hospital and the retrospective study for the coinfection of HIVAg, HIV-Ab, HCV-Ab, HBsAg and VDRL were performed [9]. According to this work, HIV-Ab was often coexistent with HBsAg and/or HCV-Ab in blood donor of Vajira Hospital [9].

1. Respiratory Tract Infection

1.1 Tuberculosis

Tuberculosis is present in every third HIV-positive person in the world. Therefore, HIV infection is considered the most evident risk factor for primary tuberculosis or relapse of latent tubercular infection [10]. Pulmonary tuberculosis is the most frequent clinical presentation in HIV-positive individuals, although the frequency of extrapulmonary tuberculosis is increasing with the CD4+ count reduction [10]. In Thailand, tuberculosis is also a very important health problem for HIV-infected cases. There are many reports on this topic, which are presented in Table 3.

1.2 Pneumocystis carinii pneumonia

In the past *Pneumocystis carinii* is classified as a protozoan but recent studies of DNA homology suggest that it is a fungus. It has two major forms, the "cyst" form and the "trophozoite" form. Both could be found in infected organs. Pneumocystis carinii pneumonia occurs at some point in the course of illness in approximately 85% of patients with AIDS [17]. Because of the frequency of Pneumocystis carinii pneumonia and because it is readily treatable, prompt, accurate, and efficient diagnostic schemes are extremely important [17]. The clinical presentation is generally characterized by fever, nonproductive cough, and shortness of breath [17]. Such symptoms in a patient from a recognized HIV transmission category should prompt a diagnostic evaluation to identify Pneumocystis carinii or other opportunistic infections [17]. In Thailand, Pneumocystis carini pneumonia is another important lung infection for HIV-infected cases. There are many reports on this topic which will be presented in Table 4.

Table 3. Reports on tuberculosis on HIV patients in Thailand

Authors	Details
Chuchottavorn et al. [11]	This is an early report on tuberculosis in Thai HIV infected cases. During the first six months of 1989, there were 456 new bacteriological proved tuberculosis patients in the Bangkok Central Chest Clinic, Tuberculosis Division [11]. All of these patients were tested to prove a possible infection of HIV by detecting the corresponding antibody in the serum [11].
Punnotok et al. [12]	This retropective study was made on the 40 male pulmonary tuberculosis patients who were intravenous drug users and found positive for HIV infection [12]. All were former prison inmates mostly in the age group of 20-40 years with the history of 1-10 years of addiction [12]. Chest radiographic picture showed mostly advanced disease with cavitation in 24 (60 %), similar to non-addict, HIV-negative patients of the same age group, but different from those as reported in other countries which mainly showed disseminated pattern and more hilar adenopathy [12].
Hongniamthong et al. [13]	In this work, Central Chest Hospital, Bangkok, conducted a study to evaluate the prevalence of HIV in new tuberculosis patients for a one-year period [13]. According to this work, there was no difference in chest X-ray appearance between the seronegative and seropositive groups in the aspect of cavitation [13]. The mean tuberculin reaction of the seropositive group was 20.2 mm lower than that of the study group, which was 22.3 mm significantly [13]. However, all of the seropositive group had tuberculin reaction greater than 10 mm [13]. The sputum smear positive rates, according to the first four days of examination, in the seropositive group and the sernonegative group were 58.6 and 34.1, respectively; only seropositive patients without full-blown AIDS had chest X-ray, tuberculin reaction and sputum smear positive rates not different from usual tuberculosis patients [13].
Bunjong [14]	From April 1, 1992 to September 30, 1994, the Tuberculosis Clinic of Singburi Hospital completed a project to study HIV infections in tuberculosis patients [14]. It was found that the HIV infection rate in 59 pulmonary tuberculosis patients whose sputum AFB were positive (infectious cases) was 6.78%. HIV infection in all new cases of pulmonary tuberculosis was 7.23% [14].
Chaimanee et al. [15]	This study was aimed to determine survival of HIV-positive tuberculosis patients compared to HIV-negative patients [15]. Through retrospective review of TB registry data of Chiang Rai Regional Hospital from October 1989 to June 1994, 1465 cases of tuberculosis patients were found, of whom 351 cases, or 24.0%, were HIV-infected. HIV-positive patients tended to be male, young, single, lowland Thai, and experiencing extrapulmonary tuberculosis, compared with HIV-negative tuberculosis patients [15]. At the end of 12 months after diagnosis, HIV-positive patients had a survival rate of 35.07%, contrast to 86.64 % in HIV-negative patients [15]. The overall probability of dying within the first 12 months after diagnosis of HIV-positive tuberculosis patients was 6.80 times as high as that of HIV-negative cases [15].
Wiriyakitjar et al. [16]	This study was aimed to determine survival of HIV-positive tuberculosis patients compared to HIV-negative patients [15]. Through retrospective review of TB registry data of Chiang Rai Regional Hospital from October 1989 to June 1994, 1465 cases of tuberculosis patients were found, of whom 351 cases or 24.0 % were HIV-infected. HIV-positive patients tended to be male, young, single, lowland Thai, and experiencing extrapulmonary tuberculosis, as compared with HIV-negative tuberculosis

Table 4. Teports on *Pneumocystis carini* pneumonia in HIV-infected patients in Thailand

Authors	Details
Himaku et al. [18]	The aim of this study is to investigate the feasibility of the conventional Papanicolaou stain in diagnosing Pneumocystis carinii pneumonia in patients with HIV infection in comparison with the special stain, Grocott modified Gomori's methenamine silver [18]. According to this work, there was no significant difference in the frequency of detection between both methods [18]. Therefore, the Papanicolaou technique, which is used routinely in the cytology laboratory, can be used for the simple and rapid initial diagnosis of Pneumocystis carinii pneumonia in bronchial washing/bronchoalveolar lavage specimens [18].
Mingvanish [19]	At Saraburi Hospital, from January 1989 to December 1992, there were 17,766 mothers who gave birth, 80 anti HIV positive mothers were included [19]. In thai period, only 4 cases of Pneumocystis carini pneumonia had been reported in HIV infants born to anti HIV positive mothers at this hospital. All cases presented with symptoms of pneumonia and bilateral bronchopneumonia by chest X-ray [19].
Vongsivavilas and Yenrudi [20]	The objective of this to study histopathologic features of Pneumocystis carini pneumonia in Thai patients with AIDS and address an outstanding issue related to pathologic diagnosis [20]. According to this work, the non-specific findings of interstitial fibrosis and/or interstitial pneumonitis were found in all patients. Intra-alveolar foamy exudate was the most common specific change in Pneumocystis carini pneumonia and was found in 49/54 (90.70 %) [20].
Wiwanitkit [21]	Wiwanitkit studied of the cost-effectiveness of three staining methods for identification of Pneumocystis carinii in bronchoalveolar lavage fluid.

1.3 Nocardiosis

Infections caused by *Nocardia* species are uncommon and have a wide variety of clinical manifestations in immunocompetent and immunocompromised patients [22]. The diagnosis of nocardiosis can easily be missed because there are no characteristic symptoms [22]. Although it is not of great concern as an AIDS-associated infection, the nonspecific clinical presentation in these patients might be confused with other lung infections such as tuberculosis [23]. The mortality rate can be as high as 60% [23]. In Thailand, there are also some reports on nocardiosis in HIV infected cases as shown in Table 5.

2. Neurological Infection

2.1 Toxoplasmosis

Toxoplasmosis is a common parasitic zoonosis and an important cause of abortions, mental retardation, encephalitis, blindness, and death worldwide [26–27]. Central nervous system is an important form of toxoplasmosis that is frequently detected as fatal infection in

HIV- infected patients [28]. In Thailand, there are few reports on toxoplasmosis in HIV infected cases [29–30].

Table 5. Reports on nocardiosis in HIV infected patients in Thailand

Authors	Details
Panitsuk [24]	The first case of pulmonary nocardiosis in HIV infected patient in Thailand was reported in this article [24]. The patient, a 32-year-old farmer, was admitted because of fever, chest pain and shortness of breath for one month. During admission, chest radiography and ultrasonography revealed loculated pleural effusion [24].
Karnkawinpong [25]	Pulmonary nocardiosis in HIV seropositive patients, Supprasitthiprasong Hospital was reported [25]. From January 1996 to March 1998, 25 HIV seropositive patients with pulmonary nocardiosis were diagnosed [25]. Modified acid-fast staining of sputum of all patients revealed branching filamentous, beaded microorganisms. Co-existing opportunistic infections were found in 16 cases (64%) with pulmonary tuberculosis being the most common (44 %) [25]. In this series, 7 cases (28 %) expired [25].

2.2 Cryptococcosis

Cryptococcus neoformans is an important fungal pathogen causing invasive infection [31]. Cryptococcosis is the most common neurological opportunistic infection in HIV infected patients. The choice of treatment depends on sites of infection and the patient's immune status [31]. Use of appropriate antifungal agents decreases mortality significantly, but requires continued therapy and long-term maintenance to prevent relapses [31]. The use of liposomal amphotericin B (L Amp B) has overcome some of the difficulties usually found in this setting [31]. According to the guideline of Infectious Diseases Society of America, among patients with HIV infection and cryptococcal meningitis, induction therapy with amphotericin B (0.7-1 mg/kg/d) plus flucytosine (100 mg/kg/d for 2 weeks) followed by fluconazole (400 mg/d) for a minimum of 10 weeks is the treatment of choice [32]. After 10 weeks of therapy, the fluconazole dosage may be reduced to 200 mg/d, depending on the patient's clinical status. Fluconazole should be continued for life [32]. In Thailand, there are also some reports on cryptococcosis in HIV infected cases as shown in Table 6.

3. Skin Infection

3.1 Penicillosis

Penicilliosis marneffei, a common mycosis among HIV infected patients living in Southeast Asia, has been recently suggested for inclusion in the surveillance case definition [36]. At present, disseminated Penicillium marneffei infection is a common opportunistic condition among HIV-infected patients in many regions in Southeast Asia, especially northern region of Thailand. Infections with *Penicillium marneffei* were rare in the past, but infections with this dimorphic fungus have increased with the endemic of HIV infection in the region [36]. *Penicilliosis marneffei* can cause two clinical types of the disease; focal and fatal progressive, disseminated infections, characterized by a variety of symptoms which can mimic those of other diseases [36–37]. For diagnosis, direct smears from skin lesion and lymphnode is usaully positive for yeast form of fungus suggestive of *Histoplasma capsulatum* but with binary fission instead of budding [38].

Table 6. Important reports on cryptococcosis in HIV-infected patients in Thailand

Authors	Details
Manosuthi et al. [33]	The objective of this work is to compare the MICs of Fluconazole and amphotericin B against isolates of *Cryptococcus neoformans* obtained from the cerebroSpinal fluid; and clinical outcomes of HIV-infected patients diagnosed with cryptococcal meningitis [33]. According to this work, the MICs of fluconzaole and amphotericin B against cerebropinal fluid isolates of *Cryptococcus neoformans* and clinical outcomes between HIV-infected patients who receive or did not receive fluconazole prophylaxis are not different [33].
Pancharoen et al. [34]	Pancharoen et al reported 8 children with cryptococcosis from King Chulalongkorn Memorial Hospital from 1991 to 2000 [34]. Five patients were older than five years [34]. The two common underlying diseases were HIV/AIDS (5 cases) and systemic lupus erythematosus (2 cases) [34]. Seven cases had been observed in the past four years, four of these in 2000 [34]. One patient developed disseminated disease and two patients died [34]. This report implies importance of central nervous system cryptococcosis in pediatric group [34].
Paoin [35]	This is another report of pediatric central nervous system cryptococcosis [35]. In this case, a thirteen-year-old boy with AIDS was admitted because of severe headache [35]. The patient developed rapid deteriolation of consciousness, dyspnea, cyanosis, seizure, shock, pulmonary hemorrhage and expired within 24 hours [35]. Numerous cryptococcus was recoverd from cerebrospinal fluid and lung necropsy [35].

3.2 Histoplasmosis

Histoplasmosis is another common skin infection in HIV infected patients. It is caused by dimorphic fungus *Histoplasma capsulatum*. Briefly, disseminated histoplasmosis was uncommon prior to the AIDS epidemic, and cutaneous eruption rarely was seen [39]. Since the onset of the worldwide AIDS epidemic, histoplasmosis has become a more common opportunistic fungal infection and should be considered in the differential diagnosis of mucocutaneous lesions in patients with AIDS in endemic areas [39]. In Thailand, there are also some reports on histoplasmosis in HIV infected cases as shown in Table 7.

Table 7. Important reports on histoplasmosis in HIV infected patients in Thailand

Authors	Details
Chirachanakul [40]	Chirachanakul reported that carbon dioxide laser could be used to ablate the epidermal layer of this lesion to identify the underlying pathogenic yeast cells by skin smear method [40]. Chirachanakul proposed that this new method was safe and effective for diagnosis of this opportunistic fungal infection in HIV infected individuals [40].
Wiwanitkit and Chaiwong [41]	Wiwanitkit and Chaiwong reported the possibility in using blood smear examination for disseminated histoplasmosis in HIV seropositive patients [41].

3.3 Candidiasis

Candidiasis is a common infection in immunocompromised host, not onlt for HIV infection. In HIV infection, oral candidiasis is an important finding. Although some patients are asymptomatic, progression of the disease may occur leading to esophageal candidiasis. Fluconazole resistant candidiasis has been reported in several international studies. Considering the recent report on skin disorder among Thai HIV-infected subjects, oral candidiasis (54.17%) was the most common opportunistic skin infections [42].

4. Gastrointestinal Infections

One of the major health problems among HIV-infected patients is the intestinal parasite infestations [43]. It can be seen that intestinal helminth infestation in HIV-infected patients is common [43]. However, the reported prevalence is usually similar to those of non HIV-infected patients in the same setting [43]. The infestations are ordinary not opportunistic, hence, thus usually show no correlation to immune status of the patients [43]. The suppression of immunity due to HIV infection shows no significant role in increasing the intestinal helminth infestations. On the other hand, having occult intestinal helminth infestations does also not worsen the outcome of HIV infection [43]. Concerning the clinical manifestation, most of the helminth infestations are asymptomatic and the diagnosis is usually based on the stool examination [43]. In Thailand, there are also some reports on histoplasmosis in HIV infected cases as shown in Table 8.

Conclusion

It can be shown that opportunistic infection is important in coping with HIV-infected cases in Thailand. In addition, practitioners who deal with patients from Thailand and nearby tropical countries should be aware of the importance of tropical infections as opportunistic infections in HIV-infected cases in Thailand.

Table 8. Reports on intestinal parasite infestations in HIV-infected patients in Thailand

Authors	Details
Wiwanitkit [44]	A study of stool samples from 60 Thai HIV-infected patients with different immune status was performed at King Chulalongkorn Memorial Hospital, Thailand [44]. Each patient was examined for CD4 count and screened for diarrheal symptoms [44]. The prevalence of intestinal parasitic infection among the HIV-infected patients in this study was 50% [44]. Non-opportunistic intestinal parasite infections such as hookworms, *Opisthorchis viverrini* and *Ascaris lumbricoides* were commonly found in HIV-infected people regardless of immune status with or without diarrheal symptoms [44]. Opportunistic intestinal parasites such as *Cryptosporidium, Isospora belli,* microsporidia and *Strongyloides stercoralis* infection were significantly more frequent in the low immunity group with diarrhea [44].
Saksirisampant et al. [45]	The prevalence of *Cryptosporidium* in 156 HIV-infected Thai patients who had acute diarrheal illness at Bamrasnaradura Infectious Diseases Hospital was studied [45]. This cross-sectional study was performed from March to August in year 2001. The patients ranged in age from 1 month to 65 years old [45]. A stool sample from each subject was stained to find the oocysts by modified Ziehl Nelson carbolfuchsin staining [45]. According to the study, a diagnosis of *Cryptosporidium parvum* infection was found in 20 patients (11 males and 9 females) [45]. The prevalence of cryptosporidiosis in the present series was 12.8% (10.0% in males and 19.1% in females) [45].
Wiwanitkit,and Srisupanant [46]	Cryptosporidiosis occurrence in anti-HIV-seropositive patients attending a sexually transmitted diseases clinic, Thailand in the era of highly active antiretroviral therapy (HAART) was reported [46]. It can be seen that HAART significantly changed the epidemiological pattern of cryptosporidiosis pattern in HIV-infected patients [46].
Wiwanitkit [47]	Microsporidiosis occurrence in anti-HIV-seropositive patients attending a sexually transmitted disease clinic, Thailand in the era of highly active antiretroviral therapy (HAART) was reported [47]. It can be seen that HAART significantly changed the epidemiological pattern of microsporidiosis pattern in HIV-infected patients [47].
Wiwanitkit and Srisupanant [48]	The pattern of intestinal parasite infestations in HIV infected patients was analyzed according to sexual behavior [48].

References

[1] Visitkijakan V. Prevalence of HIV in pregnant women in Bamrasnaradura Hospital prenatal clinic *Commun Dis J.* 1993; 19(2): 94-101.

[2] Menakanit A, Yossing R. Prevalence survey of HIV infection in pregnant women in Udornthani Hospital. *4/2 Reg Med J.* 1992; 4(2): 7-17.

[3] Sutheeravute T. The prevalence of hepatitis B virus, syphilis and human immunodeficiency virus infection in pregnant women in Samutsakhon Hospital. *J Samutsakhon Hosp.* 1992; 6(2): 132-1400.

[4] Jirapinyo M, Petchclai B, Phiromsawat S. Prevalence of positive anti-HIV in pregnant women at Ramathibodi Hospital. J Med *Assoc* Thai. 1991; 74(12): 653-657

[5] Chaiworapongsa T, Leelapattana B. Prevalence and characters of pregnant women with anti-HIV at Pramongkutklao Hospital R Thai *Army Med J.* 1993; 47(1-2) : 40-52.

[6] Kuanhin K. Prevalence of HIV infections among pregnant women in Nakhon Si Thammarat, Thailand, 1995-1996. *J Health Sci.* 1997; 6(1) : 11-19.

[7] Piyapromdee S. nce of Anemia, Syphilitic, HBV and HIV infections in pregnant women attending ANC unit at Maharat Nakhon Ratchasima Hospital . Maharat Nakhon Ratchasima Hosp Med Bull. 1994; 18(2): 153-165.

[8] Wattanachote A. Prevalence of HIV infection among blood donors at Rajavithi Hospital. Rajavithi Hosp. 1991; 1(3-4) : 29-44.

[9] Archavarungson N. The coexistent prevalence of transfusion transmitted diseaes in donated blood in Vajira Hospital. *Vajira Med J.* 1999; 43(3) : 211-217.

[10] Dabrowska MM, Pogorzelska J, Parfieniuk A, Siwak E, Wiercińska-Drapało A. Tuberculosis and HIV infection--main diagnostic and therapeutic problems. Pol Merkur Lekarski. 2007 Sep;23(135):212-4.

[11] Chuchottavorn C, Buranajaru B, Panyatungsakul P, Likanonsakul S. Prevalence of human immunodeficiency virus infection in Thai tuberculosis patients. *Thai J Tuberc Chest Dis.* 1989; 10(3): 149-156.

[12] Punnotok J, Subhannachart P, Chaisuksuwan R. Pulmonary tuberculosis among intravenous drug users with human immunodeficiency virus infection. *Thai J Tuberc Chest Dis.* 1991; 12(1): 15-24.

[13] Hongniamthong P, Chuchotethaworn C, Punnothok J, Chakorn T, Chaisooksuwan R. Prevalence of HIV infection in tuberculosis patients of Central Chest Hospital. *Commun Dis J.*1991; 17(2): 77-88.

[14] Bunjong V. HIV infection in tuberculosis patients. *Saraburi Hosp Med J.* 1997; 19(3) : 199-211

[15] Chaimanee B, Panich V, Khuntipong P, Uthaivorawit W, Yanai H, Sawanpanyalert P. Survival during the first year after diagnosis of HIV-positive and HIV-negative tuberculosis patients in Chiang Rai. *Thai J Tuberc Chest Dis.* 1997; 15(4): 237-243.

[16] Wiriyakitjar D, Na Bhuket TR, Rienthong D, Kowathana K. Surveillance of HIV infection among tuberculosis patients in Bangkok Central Chest Clinic. *Thai AIDS J.*1995; 4(1) : 14-19.

[17] Hopewell PC. Pneumocystis carinii pneumonia: diagnosis. *J Infect Dis.* 1988 Jun;157(6):1115-9.

[18] Himakun L, Chongrak C, Thongsri W, Mitchai J. The diagnosis of Pneumocystis carinii pneumonia in patients with HIV positive in cytology laboratory. *Srinagarind Med J.* 1997; 9(4): 142-147.

[19] Mingvanish S. Pneumocystis carinii pneumonia in infants born to anti HIV positive mothers. *J Med Assoc Thai.* 1993; 76(11): 641-646.

[20] Vongsivavilas Y, Yenrudi S. Histologic Features of Pneumocystis carinii pneumonia in 54 Thai AIDS patients. *Chula Med J.* 2004 ; 48(8): 539-551.

[21] Wiwanitkit V. Study of the cost-effectiveness of three staining methods for identification of Pneumocystis carinii in bronchoalveolar lavage fluid. *Trop Doct.* 2005 Jan;35(1):23-5.

[22] Agterof MJ, van der Bruggen T, Tersmette M, ter Borg EJ, van den Bosch JM, Biesma DH. Nocardiosis: a case series and a mini review of clinical and microbiological features. *Neth J Med.* 2007 Jun;65(6):199-202.

[23] Márquez-Diaz F, Soto-Ramirez LE, Sifuentes-Osornio J. Nocardiasis in patients with HIV infection. *AIDS Patient Care STDS*. 1998 Nov;12(11):825-32.

[24] Panitsuk W. Pulmonary nocardiosis associated with AIDS : a case report. Reg 7 *Med J.* 1993; 12(2): 109-112.

[25] Karnkawinpong O. Pulmonary nocardiosis in HIV seropositive patients, Supprasitthiprasong Hospital 1997-1998. *Thai J Tuberc Chest Dis*. 1988; 19(4) : 241-249.

[26] Pavesio CE, Lightman S. Toxoplasma gondii and ocular toxoplasmosis: pathogenesis. *Br J Ophthalmol*. 1996 Dec;80(12):1099-107.

[27] Klaren VN, Kijlstra A. Toxoplasmosis, an overview with emphasis on ocular involvement. *Ocul Immunol Inflamm*. 2002 Mar;10(1):1-26.

[28] Desmonts G._Central nervous system toxoplasmosis. *Pediatr Infect Dis J.* 1987 Sep;6(9):872-3.

[29] Wattanarungkowit P, Sujitranooch B. CT findings of toxoplasmic encephalitis in *AIDS. Thammasat Med J.* 2001 Feb-May; 1(2): 1-12.

[30] Nunrungroj W, Charoenhirunyingyos S, Wanachiwanawin D, Mahakittikun V, Chaisewikul R. Cerebral toxoplasmosis in AIDS patients : clinical manifestations and laboratory diagnosis. *Siriraj Hosp Gaz*. 2002; 54(6): 330-337.

[31] Subramanian S, Mathai D. Clinical manifestations and management of cryptococcal infection. *J Postgrad Med*. 2005;51 Suppl 1:S21-6.

[32] Saag MS, Graybill RJ, Larsen RA, Pappas PG, Perfect JR, Powderly WG, Sobel JD, Dismukes WE. Practice guidelines for the management of cryptococcal disease. Infectious Diseases Society of America. *Clin Infect Dis*. 2000 Apr;30(4):710-8.

[33] Manosuthi W, Sungkanuparph S, Thongyen S, Chumpathat N, Eampokalap B, Thawornwan U, Foongladda S. Antifungal susceptibilities of cryptococcus neoformans cerebrospinal fluid isolates and clinical outcomes of cryptococcal meningitis in HIV-infected patients with/without fluconazole prophylaxis. *J Med Assco Thai*. 2006; 89(6): 795-802.

[34] Pancharoen C, Chindamporn A, Thisyakorn U. Childhood cryptococcosis : an increasing problem in the era of AIDS. *J Med Assoc Thai.* 2001 Jun;84 Suppl 1:S86-90.

[35] Paoin R. Rapidly fatal cryptococcal infection in a 13-year-old AIDS patient. *J Health Sci.* 1999; 8(2): 193-201.

[36] Nittayananta W. Penicilliosis marneffei: another AIDS defining illness in Southeast Asia. *Oral Dis.* 1999 Oct;5(4):286-93.

[37] Kullavanijaya P. Penicilliosis in AIDS. *J Dermatol.* 2001 Nov;28(11):667-70.

[38] Sirivongrangson P, Timpatanapong P. Unusual cutaneous eruption of penicilliosis marneffei in AIDS. *Thai J Dermatol*. 1988; 4(1): 84.

[39] Paul AY, Aldrich S, Scott RS, Ellis MW. Disseminated histoplasmosis in a patient with AIDS: case report and review of the literature. *Cutis*. 2007 Oct;80(4):309-12.

[40] Chirachanakul P. Carbon dioxide laser-assisted epidermal ablation increases the yield of skin smear for the diagnosis of disseminated histoplasmosis in HIV-infected patient : A preliminary study. *Thai J Dermatol*. 2005; 21(2): 76-81.

[41] Wiwanitkit V, Chaiwong T. Blood smear examination for disseminated histoplasmosis in 50 HIV seropositive patients in Chulalongkorn Hospital. *Srinagarind Med J*. 2003 ; 18(1): 27-29.

[42] Wiwanitkit V. Prevalence of dermatological disorders in Thai HIV-infected patients correlated with different CD4 lymphocyte count statuses: a note on 120 cases. *Int J Dermatol*. 2004 Apr;43(4):265-8.

[43] Wiwanitkit V. Intestinal parasite infestation in HIV infected patients. *Curr HIV Res*. 2006 Jan;4(1):87-96.

[44] Wiwanitkit V. inal parasitic infections in Thai HIV-infected patients with different immunity status.*BMC Gastroenterol*. 2001;1:3.

[45] Saksirisampant W, Eampokalap B, Rattanasrithong M, Likanonsakul S, Wiwanitkit V, Nasingkarn A, Denmasae N. A prevalence of Cryptosporidium infections among Thai HIV-infected patients. *J Med Assoc Thai*. 2002 Jun;85 Suppl 1:S424-8.

[46] Wiwanitkit V, Srisupanant M. Cryptosporidiosis occurrence in anti-HIV-seropositive patients attending a sexually transmitted diseases clinic, *Thailand. Trop Doct*. 2006 Jan;36(1):64

[47] Wiwanitkit V. Antiretroviral therapy and intestinal microsporidiosis in Thai HIV infected patients. *Parasite*. 2007 Sep;14(3):252.

[48] Wiwanitkit V, Srisupanant M. Opportunistic intestinal parasite infection and mode of sexual intercourse of HIV-infected patients in the era of HAART。 *Sexual Disabil*. 2006; 24(4): 213-215.

In: AIDS- Related Opportunistic Infections
Editor: Claudia D. Galanda

ISBN: 978-1-60692-144-9

Chapter VIII

The Prevention of AIDS-Related Malignancies

Justin Stebbing*, Tom Powles, Robert Glassman[1], Vanessa Marvin and Mark Bower

The Department of Immunology, Division of Investigative Science, Faculty of Medicine, Imperial College of Science, Technology and Medicine, The Chelsea and Westminster Hospital, London,United Kingdom

[1] Division of Hematology-Oncology, Weill Medical College of Cornell University, New York, New York, USA

Abstract

The immune surveillance hypothesis of cancer emerged during the twentieth century but until recently there have been few clinical examples of immunoprevention of malignancy. The worldwide epidemic of the human immunodeficiency virus (HIV) represent the most striking example of genome emergence, transmission and expansion. Concomitantly, the field of anti-retroviral therapy has witnessed remarkable progress and there are now over fifteen approved therapeutic agents for treatment of this pathogen that once caused a uniformly fatal illness. With longer term follow-up, we also observe that the anti-retroviral induced maintenance of immunocompetence, also prevents common HIV-related malignancies. This is discussed below with specific reference to effective anti-retroviral therapy preventing both Kaposi's sarcoma and non Hodgkin's lymphoma in advanced HIV disease.

Keywords: cancer; tumors; HAART; immunotherapy

* Address for correspondence: j.stebbing@imperial.ac.uk

Historical Perspectives on Immunoprevention

William Coley, a surgeon first noticed at the turn of the 20th century that cancer patients who developed bacterial infections had tumors that became necrotic [1,2]. In the hope of curing cancer, Coley started injecting cancer patients with supernatants derived from certain bacterial cultures. These injections termed "Coley's toxins," showed some success in producing necrosis of tumors but had negative side effects. Soon after, Paul Ehrlich and Ilya Ilyich Mechnikov (Figure 1) were awarded the Nobel prize for their hypothesis of the immune surveillance theory of cancer in which they suggested that the immune system continually 'removes' tumours that arise spontaneously. Their theories lay largely dormant until the emergence of allogeneic transplant medicine in the 1960s.

The first renal transplant was performed between identical twins by Joseph Murray at Boston's Bringham Hospital in 1953. The development of azathioprine by George Hitchins and Gertrude Elion ten years later enabled successful allogeneic transplantation and began an era of transplantation medicine dependent upon iatrogenic immunosuppression. The allogeneic organ transplant recipients who received immunosuppressant therapy were found to be prone to post-transplantation lymphoproliferative diseases and other tumours including Kaposi's sarcoma and it was noticed later that these tumours regressed on cessation of immunosuppression [3-6].

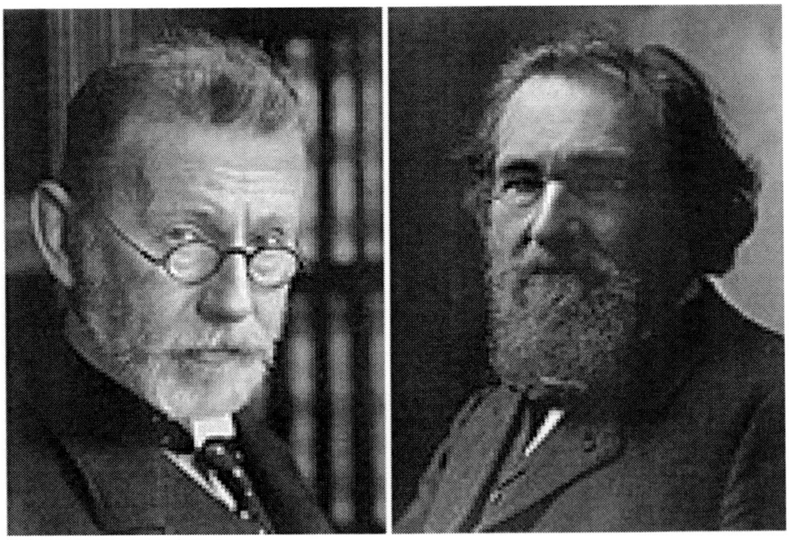

Figure 1. The Nobel prize in physiology or medicine was awarded equally between Ilya Ilyich Mechnikov (left, 1845 – 1916, Institut Pasteur, Paris) and Paul Ehrlich (right, 1854 – 1915, Goettingen University and Königliches Institut für experimentelle Therapie Frankfurt). They coined the term 'magic bullets' and starting off with an arsenic compound, atoxyl, they synthesised Salvarsan (dihydroxydiaminoarsenobenzenedihydrochloride). Salvarsan was first tried on rabbits that had been infected with syphilis and then on patients with the dementia associated with the final stages of the disease. Astonishingly, several of these 'terminal' patients recovered after treatment with Salvarsan. More testing revealed that Salvarsan was actually more successful if administered during the early stages of syphilis. Salvarsan (1909) and Neosalvarsan (1912) retained their role as the most effective drugs for treating syphilis until the widespread availability of antibiotics in the 1940s.

At this time, Klein *et al.* demonstrated the extraordinary phenomenon that one could immunise against tumours in the same manner as was being performed with remarkable success against polio and smallpox [7,8]. A decade later it was determined that Coley's toxins contained bacterial endotoxin which stimulated immune cells to secrete a substance that has an anti-tumor effect [9]. Further research on this substance showed that it had a direct necrosis effect on tumor cells and thus gained its name--tumor necrosis factor [10].

In 1983, the New York Times headline "Rare cancer seen in 41 homosexuals" formed part of the events that heralded the onset of the human immunodeficiency virus type-1 (HIV) epidemic [11]. The increased risk of cancers in patients with iatrogenic, primary or acquired immunosuppression has firmly established a role for the immune system in the control of cancer [12]. In particular, a large number of cancers including Kaposi's sarcoma (KS) and non Hodgkin's lymphoma (NHL) are observed at a frequency of greater than 100 times in HIV infected individuals, compared to non-infected controls [13-16]. However, the prevention of AIDS-related malignancies has not utilised host immunity but rather, focused on attacking the virus that causes AIDS.

Highly Active Anti-Retroviral Therapy

One year following this New York Times headline, the human immunodeficiency virus (HIV) was identified as the causative agent of the acquired immunodeficiency syndrome (AIDS) [17]. The rapid elucidation of the crystal structures of its protease [18,19] and reverse transcriptase [20,21] has led to the development of highly active anti-retroviral therapy (HAART), currently available for less than one million of the 60 million HIV-1 infected people worldwide [22]. HAART controls viral replication, allows for immune restoration and numerous studies that have recruited many thousands of patients have shown that it reduces mortality and morbidity [23,24]. Now, almost every part of the life-cycle of HIV has been targeted including capsid assembly and fusion with the host cell membrane (Figure 2). HAART now consists of either a protease inhibitor and/ or a non nucleoside reverse trascriptase inhibitor with a nucleoside analogue backbone [25].

In established market economies, HAART has led to a reduced incidence of KS and other AIDS-associated malignancies such as non-Hodgkin's lymphoma that are often due to secondary viral infections [26-28]. For KS, HAART can lead to resolution of individual lesions [29,30] although this has not been observed for NHL.

A common feature of malignancies in the setting of HIV is the role of other viruses, namely Kaposi's sarcoma-associated herpesvirus (KSHV), Epstein Barr virus (EBV) and human papillomavirus (HPV). Figure 3 demonstrates the interplay between the immune system, infection and cancer. In advanced HIV infection, immunoparesis results in either overwhelming infection with secondary viruses or, in most cases we observe, long-lasting infection during which cellular transformation occurs.

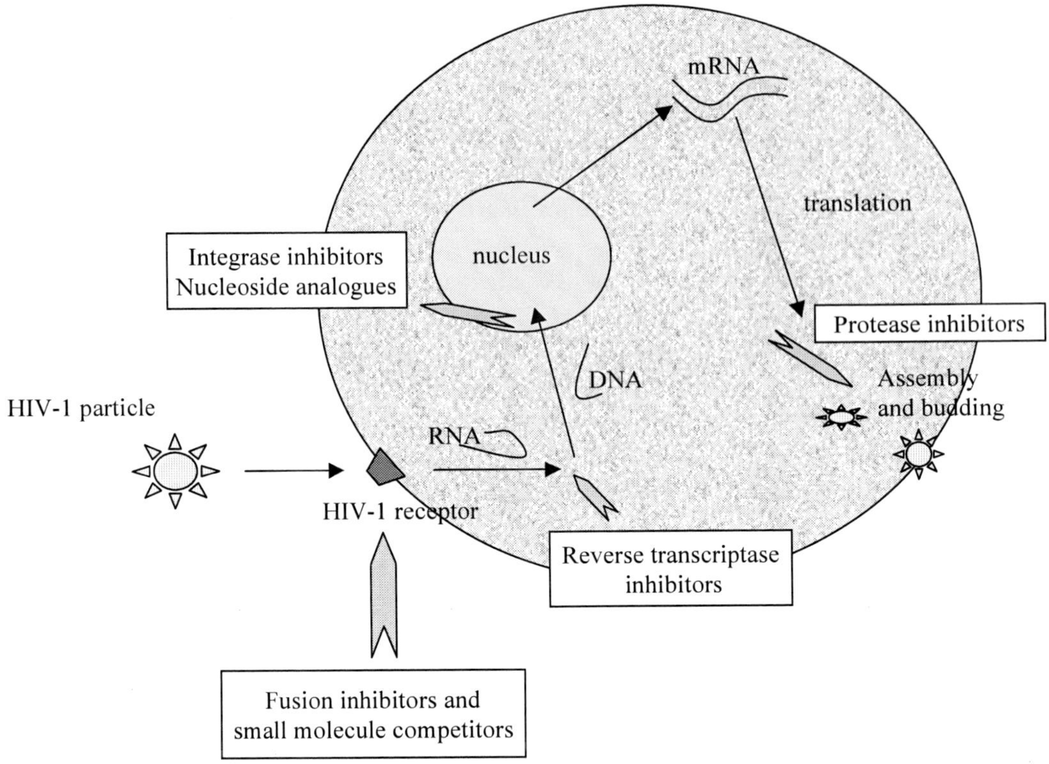

Figure 2. The life-cycle of HIV and sites of action of anti-retroviral drugs. Newer therapies include the fusion and integrase inhibitors and small molecules that compete with receptor binding of the virus. There are considerable overlaps between the immunotherapy for infectious diseases and cancer and most approaches are applicable to both situations. As viruses target conserved pathways in cellular evolution, an understanding of these facilitates an appreciation of cell cycle and apoptotic pathways, critical for carcinogenesis.

The Immunoprevention of Kaposi's Sarcoma

HAART has an established place as primary therapy for KS and there are even anecdotal reports in the literature describing complete remission of visceral KS with non-protease inhibitor based triple therapy [31,32]. We have also demonstrated a role for HAART as adjuvant therapy for KS following chemotherapy or radiotherapy. In this circumstance HAART prolongs the median time to treatment failure for KS to 1.7 years [30]. This was statistically longer than the equivalent time for the same cohort of patients before they started HAART (log rank χ^2=16.5, p<0.0001).

Prior to the development of HAART interferon-α was used as a form of non-specific immunotherapy for KS with response rates of up to 30%. The response rates were highest in patients with CD4 cell counts above 200 cells/mm^3. The use of interferon-α including pegylated forms with an increased half life to treat KS, has its origins in the management of othertumours such as renal cell carcinoma [33] and melanoma [34,35] where limited success has been reported.

Figure 3A. The response to cacrinogenic viral infection often results in the establishment of chronic infection. For many viruses such as the herpesviridae which include Epstein Barr virus, human papillomavirus and Kaposi's sarcoma-associated herpesvirus this can be entirely asymptomatic. Host factors including HLA type and receptor polymorphisms influence the outcome.

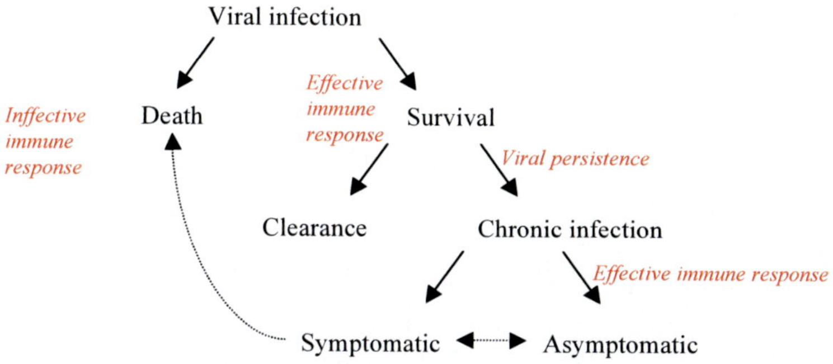

Figure 3B. The progression of HPV towards invasive carcinoma involves a sequence of events influenced by factors including viral sub-type, loss of immune control including immunodeficiency and environmental influences such as smoking. The HPV E6 and E7 proteins interact with the tumour suppressors retinoblastoma and p53 respectively leading to uncontrolled proliferation through cell cycle checkpoints.

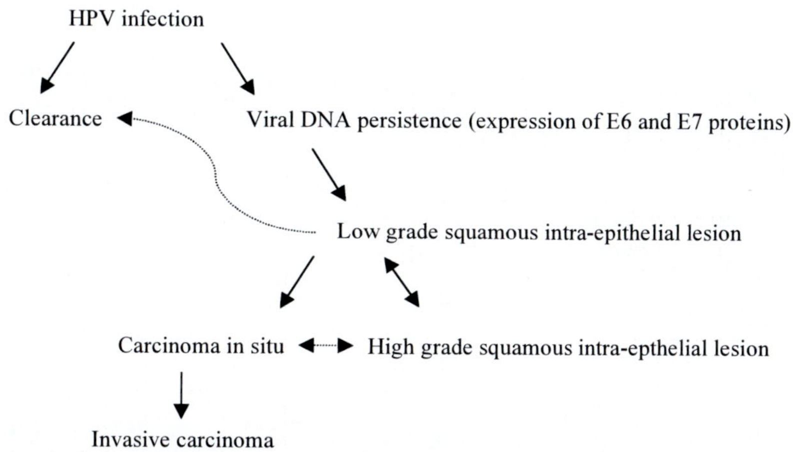

Figure 3. The different outcomes after challenge with a virus. Figure 3A. The response to cacrinogenic viral infection often results in the establishment of chronic infection. For many viruses such as the herpesviridae which include Epstein Barr virus, human papillomavirus and Kaposi's sarcoma-associated herpesvirus this can be entirely asymptomatic. Host factors including HLA type and receptor polymorphisms influence the outcome. Figure 3B. The progression of HPV towards invasive carcinoma involves a sequence of events influenced by factors including viral sub-type, loss of immune control including immunodeficiency and environmental influences such as smoking. The HPV E6 and E7 proteins interact with the tumour suppressors retinoblastoma and p53 respectively leading to uncontrolled proliferation through cell cycle checkpoints.

At the Chelsea and Westminster Hospital, we have shown a reduced incidence of KS in the HAART era and we wished to investigate whether one type of HAART may be superior to others. One seminal study compared KS chemoprevention by anti-retrovirals to determine whether this anti-KS effect was largely confined to protease inhibitors (PIs) as has been previously suggested. Multi-variate logistic regression analyses of 1204 cases of AIDS-KS seen between 1986 and 2002, found that the incidence decreased from 30 cases per thousand patient years (PY) prior to 1995 to 7.6 immediately thereafter. This was clearly co-incident with treatment using dual nucleoside analogue reverse transcriptase inhibitors. More recently, the incidence has fallen dramatically to 0.03 cases per thousand patient years, although to our surprise patients receiving non-PI based therapies had a statistically significant difference in their incidence of KS when compared with those treated with PIs: 0.2 cases per 1000 patient years (95% CI 0.02-0.12) versus 1.1 cases per 1000 patient years (95% CI 0.15-0.38) respectively (p = 0.002). This study, the first showing a decreased incidence of an AIDS-defining illness with non nucleoside reverse transcriptase inhibitor based therapy, demonstrates that non-PI based regimens are at least as effective as PI-based HAART in terms of protection against KS [36].

Figure 4 demonstrates the probability of developing KS decreases with appropriate protease inhibitor (PI) or non nucleoside reverse transcriptase inhibitor (NNRTI) containing HAART.

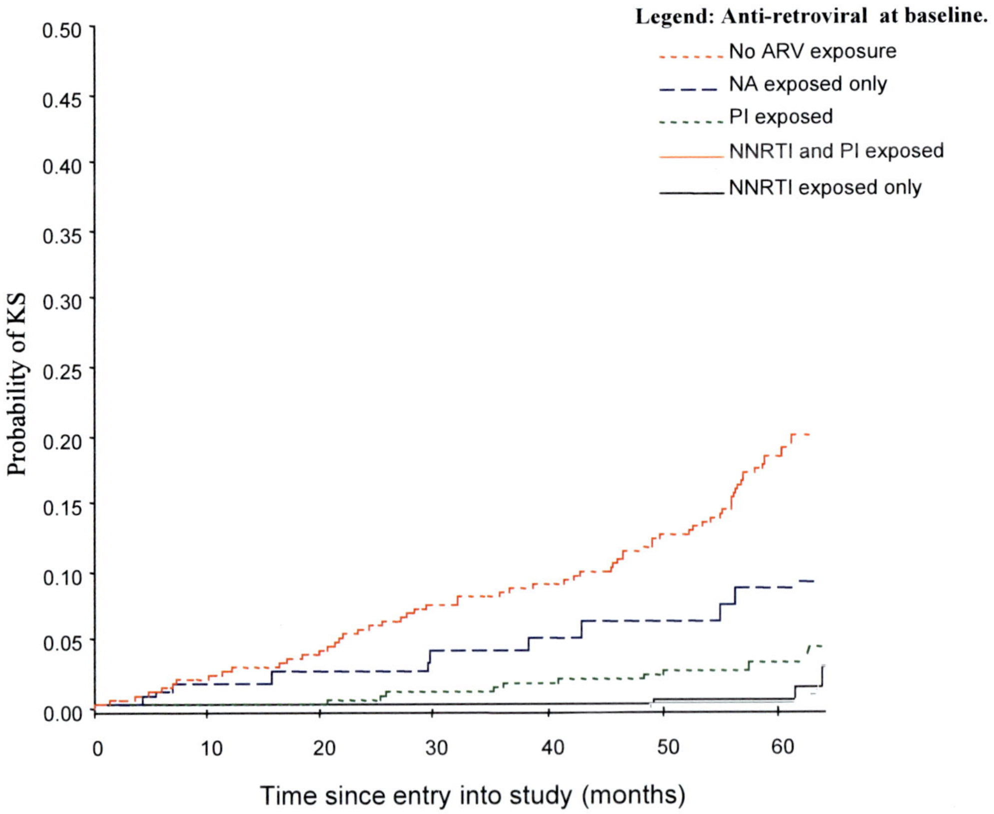

Figure 4. The probability of KS and baseline exposure to different antiretrovirals over 5 years. Almost an identical figure is observed for NHL.

Non-Specific Immune Therapy for Non Hodgin's Lymphoma

NHL has been classified as an AIDS-defining illness (ADI) following its first description at the onset of the HIV pandemic [37-40]. It remains the second commonest tumour associated with HIV-1 infection following KS, and many patients present with widespread disease; the risk of CNS involvement is also increased compared with HIV-negative counterparts [30,41].

In the multivariate analyses discussed above, we have also demonstrated that decreases in adaptive immune parameters (T and B cell counts) predispose individuals to KS and increases confer protection [42]. Innate markers (natural killer counts) appear to have a less significant role in established disease [43]. We therefore wished to establish whether NNRTI- or PI- based HAART conferred increased protection against AIDS-related NHL, and investigated changes in immune function that may protect or predispose HIV-1 infected individuals.

Using a similar logistic regression analysis as for KS, we found that NNRTI or PI-based HAART regimens and both in combination appear equally effective at protecting from NHL and the combination of two antiretroviral classes conferred significantly more protection than nucleoside analogues alone. We also confirmed as independent risk factors that increased age and low T lymphocyte counts, both CD4 and CD8, led to an increased incidence of NHL. Markers of the innate (CD16/56) and humoral (CD19) immune systems did not demonstrate significance when adjustments were made for other factors. This included sub-group analyses of patients with Burkitt's lymphoma.

The role of the immune system in the control of AIDS-related NHL is only now being established. EBV has been implicated in the aetiopathogenesis of B cell transformation for many years and both CD4 and CD8 positive T cells play significant roles in preventing viral replication [44]. We observed that at higher CD4 counts, the rate ratio of NHL was not increased at different quartiles of CD8 counts, lending credence to the importance of CD4 T cell help in the CD8 response to EBV [45,46]. The incidence and rate ratio of NHL appears greatest at lower CD4 and CD8 counts with CD4 counts exerting the greatest influence on risk.

By mimicking B-cell antigen-activation pathways, EBV enters the long-lived memory B lymphocyte pool where it evades immune elimination by severely restricting its own gene expression [47]. Higher EBV viral loads have recently been found associated with lower CD4 counts and in HIV-1 positive individuals versus controls [48-50]. In a study of HIV-1 infected children, high EBV viral burden was significantly associated with the development of malignancy, an effect modified by higher CD4 cell counts [51]. Also consistent with the data presented here, zidovudine antiretroviral therapy alone, a nucleoside analogue, did not confer a significant protective effect for either the high (OR, 0.81; 95% CI, 0.22-3.09; $p = 0.77$) or the low CD4 cell count groups (OR, 0.27; 95% CI, 0.04-1.46; $p = 0.16$). Effective HAART appears a prerequisite for prevention of both NHL and KS and sub-group analysis of specific effects of the PI ritonavir, noted to have specific anti-angiogenic properties *in vitro* [52], for KS and NHL patients do not show additional benefits [53].

As the analyses here was adjusted for time since diagnosis, it is notable that age is independent risk factor for the development of NHL, although the association became weaker in the multivariate analysis (adjusted rate ratio 1.07 in univariate analysis versus 1.02 in multivariate). HAART may be able to decelerate age-related thymic atrophy [54] and mechanisms dependent on interleukin-7 are postulated to play a role [55]. As the majority cancers are more common with age, a feature interestingly observed in large studies examining seropositivity rates of chronic infections [56,57], this was perhaps unsurprising.

Since the introduction of HAART, while a declining incidence of KS was noted within a few years, a concomitant decrease in NHL was not observed for a longer period and some studies reported no decline [41]. In one prospective European study, the incidence of AIDS-defining illnesses decreased from 30.7 per 100 patient years in 1994 to 2.5 per 100 patient years in 1998 [58]. Only NHL increased as an AIDS-defining condition during this time; 4% of patients had lymphoma as an ADI in 1994 compared with 16% in 1998. In an analysis of 23 prospective cohort studies (n = 47,936) from patients living in established market economies, a decline in the incidence of NHL was reported for the first time, from 6.2 cases per 1000 person years in 1992 to 3.6 cases per 1000 patient years in 1999 [26]. The differences in KS and NHL epidemiological features may be explained by an improvement in immune function on HAART preventing KS in the short term, with an increased duration of therapy required to prevent NHL. Supporting this hypothesis, we observed that increased B cell counts protect from KS and KS lesions may resolve with HAART alone, unlike the situation with NHL [42]. In addition, natural killer cells, first identified by their ability to lyse lymphoma cells [59,60] did not appear to have a significant role here in the multivariate analysis suggesting that their role may be limited to early events in tumorigenesis.

HPV Related Cancers

Anal and cervical cancer are thought to share aetiopathologies and both have an increasing incidence, particularly in individuals infected with HIV-1. Both are thought to arise from the progression of squamous intra-epithelial lesions to invasive cancer [61]. There is a substantial body of literature demonstrating improvements in cervical squamous intra-epithelial lesions in women successfully treated with anti-retroviral agents [62,63]. The natural history of anal intra-epithelial neoplasia has not however been established, nor has the effect of treatment with anti-retrovirals [64]. In a small cohort of gay men with anal intraepithelial neoplasia, we were unable to establish any role that 're-constitution' of the immune system using HAART resulted in regression of pre-malignant lesions [65,66].

We are no establishing whether screening of gay men for anal intra-epithelial neoplasia will be a useful modality. Data suggest that local excision followed by combined chemo and radiotherapy is an effective treatment for anal squamous carcinoma detected at an early stage. This approach is clearly not ideal, but in the long term more acceptable treatments: topical, immunomodulatory or surgical, can only be developed if there is a cohort of patients with high grade disease. We are currently conducting a double-blind placebo controlled study using the topical immune stimulant imiquimod (a toll like receptor-7 agonist) in the anal canal.

Conclusions

The first benefits of HAART were those that led to a decrease in morbidity and mortality via the prevention of opportunistic infections such as *Pneumocystis carinii pneumoniae* [23,24]. Now, we are observing protection from tumors due to, we presume, a decrease in latent opportunistic infections caused by carcinogenic viruses such as KSHV in the case of KS, EBV in the case of NHL and HPV in the case of anal and cervical cancers. HAART induced suppression of HIV viremia leading to maintenance of immune function appears critical here. The explosion of knowledge in the innate immune system and newer therapies that stimulate this (such as imiquimod) may well be critical in the 'war against cancer'.

The data we discuss also indicate that PI-sparing HAART regimens can be used in the prevention of cancer. This reduces both the toxicity and the complexity of the antiretroviral regimens, and improves long-term adherence. Such clinical data should provide reassurance to clinicians when advising patients on therapeutic options.

For the developing world, long term HAART appears a necessity to prevent both of these particular ADIs. It appears that the treatment of HIV is at least as important if not more than the selection of any subsequent chemotherapy itself. Available clinical trial data should be used to encourage the development of long-term anti-HIV strategies to manage AIDS-related lymphoma and AIDS-related KS in parts of the world where the burden is greatest [67-69].

Significantly a wide range of HAART appears protective against both NHL and KS and this is probably achieved by maintaining adequate T lymphocyte counts. Thus, the choice of anti-retrovirals as chemoprophylaxis for common neoplastic ADIs is diverse and can be considered to be 'any HAART regimen'.

References

[1] Haux J. Infection and cancer. *Lancet*. 2001;358:155-156

[2] Gresser I. A. Chekhov, M.D., and Coley's toxins. *N Engl J Med*. 1987;317:457

[3] Siegel JH, Janis R, Alper JC, Schutte H, Robbins L, Blaufox MD. Disseminated visceral Kaposi's sarcoma. Appearance after human renal homograft operation. *Jama*. 1969;207:1493-1496

[4] Myers BD, Kessler E, Levi J, Pick A, Rosenfeld JB, Tikvah P. Kaposi sarcoma in kidney transplant recipients. *Arch Intern Med*. 1974;133:307-311

[5] Penn I. Kaposi's sarcoma in organ transplant recipients: report of 20 cases. *Transplantation*. 1979;27:8-11.

[6] Euvrard S, Kanitakis J, Claudy A. Skin cancers after organ transplantation. *N Engl J Med*. 2003;348:1681-1691

[7] Klein G, Sjorgen HO, Klein E, Hellstrom KE. Demonstration of resistance against methylchol-anthrene-induced sarcomas in the primary autochth-onous host. *Cancer Research*. 1960;20:1561-1562

[8] Klein G. Tumor antigens. Annu Rev Microbiol. 1966;20:223-252

[9] Carswell EA, Old LJ, Kassel RL, Green S, Fiore N, Williamson B. An endotoxin-induced serum factor that causes necrosis of tumors. *Proc Natl Acad Sci U S A*. 1975;72:3666-3670

[10] Old LJ. Tumor necrosis factor (TNF). *Science*. 1985;230:630-632

[11] Bayer R, Oppenheimer GM. *AIDS Doctors, voices from the epidemic, an oral history*. Oxford: Oxford University Press; 2002

[12] Stebbing J, Portsmouth S, Bower M. Insights into the molecular biology and sero-epidemiology of Kaposi's sarcoma. *Current opinions in infectious diseases*. 2003;16:25-31

[13] Ledergerber B, Telenti A, Egger M. Risk of HIV related Kaposi's sarcoma and non-Hodgkin's lymphoma with potent antiretroviral therapy: prospective cohort study. *Bmj*. 1999;319:23-24

[14] Ratner L, Lee J, Tang S, Redden D, Hamzeh F, Herndier B, Scadden D, Kaplan L, Ambinder R, Levine A, Harrington W, Grochow L, Flexner C, Tan B, Straus D. Chemotherapy for human immunodeficiency virus-associated non-Hodgkin's lymphoma in combination with highly active antiretroviral therapy. *J Clin Oncol*. 2001;19:2171-2178.

[15] Otieno MW, Banura C, Katongole-Mbidde E, Johnson JL, Ghannoum M, Dowlati A, Renne R, Arts E, Whalen C, Lederman MM, Remick SC. Therapeutic challenges of AIDS-related non-Hodgkin's lymphoma in the United States and East Africa. *J Natl Cancer Inst*. 2002;94:718-732.

[16] Thirlwell C, Sarker D, Stebbing J, Bower M. Acquired immunodeficiency syndrome-related lymphoma in the era of highly active antiretroviral therapy. *Clin Lymphoma*. 2003;4:86-92

[17] Barre-Sinoussi F, Chermann J C, Rey F, Nugeyre M T, Chamaret S, Gruest J, Daugert C, Axler-Blin C, Vezinet-Brun F, Rouzioux C, Rozenbaum W, Montagnier L. Isolation of a T-lymphotropic retrovirus from a patient at risk for acquired immune deficiency syndrome (AIDS). *Science*. 1983;220:868-871

[18] Pearl LH, Taylor WR. A structural model for the retroviral proteases. *Nature*. 1987;329:351-354.

[19] Miller M, Jaskolski M, Rao JK, Leis J, Wlodawer A. Crystal structure of a retroviral protease proves relationship to aspartic protease family. *Nature*. 1989;337:576-579.

[20] Arnold E, Jacobo-Molina A, Nanni RG, Williams RL, Lu X, Ding J, Clark AD, Jr., Zhang A, Ferris AL, Clark P, et al. Structure of HIV-1 reverse transcriptase/DNA complex at 7 A resolution showing active site locations. *Nature*. 1992;357:85-89.

[21] Kohlstaedt LA, Wang J, Friedman JM, Rice PA, Steitz TA. Crystal structure at 3.5 A resolution of HIV-1 reverse transcriptase complexed with an inhibitor. *Science*. 1992;256:1783-1790.

[22] Stebbing J, Patterson S, Gotch F. New insights into the immunology and evolution of HIV. *Cell Res*. 2003;13:1-7.

[23] Palella FJ, Jr., Delaney KM, Moorman AC, Loveless MO, Fuhrer J, Satten GA, Aschman DJ, Holmberg SD. Declining morbidity and mortality among patients with advanced human immunodeficiency virus infection. HIV Outpatient Study Investigators. *N Engl J Med*. 1998;338:853-860.

[24] Hammer SM. Increasing choices for HIV therapy. *N Engl J Med.* 2002;346:2022-2023.

[25] British HIV Association (BHIVA) guidelines for the treatment of HIV-infected adults with antiretroviral therapy. *HIV Med.* 2001;2:276-313.

[26] Bosing T, Bellos F, Cremer FW, Gemmel C, Moldenhauer G, Ho AD, Goldschmidt H, Moos M. CD19+ and CD20+ B cells from the peripheral blood of patients with multiple myeloma are not infected with human herpesvirus 8. *Leukemia.* 2000;14:1330-1331

[27] Bower M, Nelson M, Portsmouth S, Mandalia S, Gazzard BG. *Falling incidence of AIDS related Kaposi's sarcoma on HAART: The protective effect of NNRTI's.* World AIDS conference. Barcelona; 2002

[28] Stebbing J, Portsmouth S, Gotch F, Gazzard B. Kaposi's sarcoma--an update. *Int J STD AIDS.* 2003;14:225-227.

[29] Jacobson LP, Yamashita TE, Detels R, Margolick JB, Chmiel JS, Kingsley LA, Melnick S, Munoz A. Impact of potent anti-retroviral therapy on the incidence of Kaposi's sarcoma and non-Hodgkin's lymphomas among HIV-1 infected individuals. Multicenter AIDS Cohort Study. *J Acquir Immune Defic Syndr.* 1999;21 Suppl 1:s34-41

[30] Bower M, Fox P, Fife K, Gill J, Nelson M, Gazzard B. Highly active anti-retroviral therapy (HAART) prolongs time to treatment failure in Kaposi's sarcoma. *Aids.* 1999;13:2105-2111.

[31] Langford A, Ruf B, Kunze R, Pohle HD, Reichart P. Regression of oral Kaposi's sarcoma in a case of AIDS on zidovudine (AZT). *Br J Dermatol.* 1989;120:709-713.

[32] Murdaca G, Campelli A, Setti M, Indiveri F, Puppo F. Complete remission of AIDS/Kaposi's sarcoma after treatment with a combination of two nucleoside reverse transcriptase inhibitors and one non-nucleoside reverse transcriptase inhibitor. *Aids.* 2002;16:304-305.

[33] Stebbing J, Benson C, Eisen T, Pyle L, Smalley K, Bridle H, Mak I, Sapunar F, Ahern R, Gore ME. The treatment of advanced renal cell cancer with high-dose oral thalidomide. *Br J Cancer.* 2001;85:953-958.

[34] Stebbing J, Gore M. Preventing relapse in melanoma. *Curr Oncol Rep.* 2000;2:205-208

[35] Brown CK, Kirkwood JM. Medical management of melanoma. *Surg Clin North Am.* 2003;83:283-322, viii

[36] Portsmouth S, Stebbing J, Gill J, Mandalia S, Bower M, Nelson M, Gazzard B. A comparison of regimens based on non-nucleoside reverse transcriptase inhibitors or protease inhibitors in preventing Kaposi's sarcoma. *Aids.* 2003;17:F17-22

[37] Ziegler JL, Drew WL, Miner RC, Mintz L, Rosenbaum E, Gershow J, Lennette ET, Greenspan J, Shillitoe E, Beckstead J, Casavant C, Yamamoto K. Outbreak of Burkitt's-like lymphoma in homosexual men. *Lancet.* 1982;2:631-633.

[38] Ziegler JL, Beckstead JA, Volberding PA, Abrams DI, Levine AM, Lukes RJ, Gill PS, Burkes RL, Meyer PR, Metroka CE, et al. Non-Hodgkin's lymphoma in 90 homosexual men. Relation to generalized lymphadenopathy and the acquired immunodeficiency syndrome. *N Engl J Med.* 1984;311:565-570.

[39] Ziegler JL, Bragg K, Abrams D, Beckstead J, Cogan M, Volberding P, Baer D, Wilkinson L, Rosenbaum E, Grant K, et al. High-grade non-Hodgkin's lymphoma in patients with AIDS. *Ann N Y Acad Sci*. 1984;437:412-419.

[40] Stebbing J, Bower M. What can oncologists learn from HIV? *Lancet Oncol*. 2003;4:438-445

[41] Matthews GV, Bower M, Mandalia S, Powles T, Nelson MR, Gazzard BG. Changes in acquired immunodeficiency syndrome-related lymphoma since the introduction of highly active antiretroviral therapy. *Blood*. 2000;96:2730-2734.

[42] Stebbing J, Gazzard B, Newsom-Davis T, Nelson M, Patterson S, Gotch F, Mandalia S, Bower M. Nadir B cell counts are significantly correlated with the risk of Kaposi's sarcoma. *Int J Cancer*. 2004;108:473-474

[43] Stebbing J, Gazzard B, Flore O, Thomas C, Benlahrech A, Mandalia S, Bower M, Gotch F, Patterson S. Natural killer cells are not infected by Kaposi's sarcoma-associated herpesvirus in vivo, and natural killer cell counts do not correlate with the risk of developing Kaposi's sarcoma. *Aids*. 2003;17:1998-2000.

[44] Amyes E, Hatton C, Montamat-Sicotte D, Gudgeon N, Rickinson AB, McMichael AJ, Callan MF. Characterization of the CD4+ T cell response to Epstein-Barr virus during primary and persistent infection. *J Exp Med*. 2003;198:903-911.

[45] Fu Z, Cannon MJ. Functional analysis of the CD4(+) T-cell response to Epstein-Barr virus: T-cell-mediated activation of resting B cells and induction of viral BZLF1 expression. *J Virol*. 2000;74:6675-6679.

[46] Yu Q, Gu JX, Kovacs C, Freedman J, Thomas EK, Ostrowski MA. Cooperation of TNF family members CD40 ligand, receptor activator of NF-kappa B ligand, and TNF-alpha in the activation of dendritic cells and the expansion of viral specific CD8+ T cell memory responses in HIV-1-infected and HIV-1-uninfected individuals. *J Immunol*. 2003;170:1797-1805.

[47] Macsween KF, Crawford DH. Epstein-Barr virus-recent advances. *Lancet Infect Dis*. 2003;3:131-140.

[48] Rickinson AB, Moss DJ. Human cytotoxic T lymphocyte responses to Epstein-Barr virus infection. Annu Rev Immunol. 1997;15:405-431

[49] Ling PD, Vilchez RA, Keitel WA, Poston DG, Peng RS, White ZS, Visnegarwala F, Lewis DE, Butel JS. Epstein-Barr virus DNA loads in adult human immunodeficiency virus type 1-infected patients receiving highly active antiretroviral therapy. *Clin Infect Dis*. 2003;37:1244-1249.

[50] Chakrabarti S, Milligan DW, Pillay D, Mackinnon S, Holder K, Kaur N, McDonald D, Fegan CD, Waldmann H, Hale G, Rickinson A, Steven N. Reconstitution of the Epstein-Barr virus-specific cytotoxic T-lymphocyte response following T-cell-depleted myeloablative and nonmyeloablative allogeneic stem cell transplantation. *Blood*. 2003;102:839-842.

[51] Pollock BH, Jenson HB, Leach CT, McClain KL, Hutchison RE, Garzarella L, Joshi VV, Parmley RT, Murphy SB. Risk factors for pediatric human immunodeficiency virus-related malignancy. *Jama*. 2003;289:2393-2399.

[52] Pati S, Pelser CB, Dufraine J, Bryant JL, Reitz MS, Jr., Weichold FF. Antitumorigenic effects of HIV protease inhibitor ritonavir: inhibition of Kaposi sarcoma. *Blood.* 2002;99:3771-3779

[53] Stebbing J, Portsmouth S, Nelson M, Mandalia S, Kandil H, Alexander N, Davies L, Brock C, Bower M, Gazzard B. The efficacy of ritonavir in the prevention of AIDS-related Kaposi's sarcoma. *Int J Cancer*. 2004;108:631-633

[54] Pido-Lopez J, Burton C, Hardy G, Pires A, Sullivan A, Gazzard B, Aspinall R, Gotch F, Imami N. Thymic output during initial highly active antiretroviral therapy (HAART) and during HAART supplementation with interleukin 2 and/or with HIV type 1 immunogen (Remune). *AIDS Res Hum Retroviruses*. 2003;19:103-109.

[55] Andrew D, Aspinall R. Il-7 and not stem cell factor reverses both the increase in apoptosis and the decline in thymopoiesis seen in aged mice. *J Immunol.* 2001;166:1524-1530.

[56] Sitas F, Carrara H, Beral V, Newton R, Reeves G, Bull D, Jentsch U, Pacella-Norman R, Bourboulia D, Whitby D, Boshoff C, Weiss R, Patel M, Ruff P, Bezwoda WR, Retter E, Hale M. Antibodies against Human Herpesvirus 8 in Black South African Patients with Cancer. *N Engl J Med*. 1999;340:1863-1871

[57] Stebbing J, Bourloulia D, Johnson M, Henderson S, Gotch F, Boshoff C. KSHV specific CTLs target Darwinian positively selected autologous epitopes within ORF-K1. *Journal of Virology*. 2003;In press

[58] Mocroft A, Vella S, Benfield TL, Chiesi A, Miller V, Gargalianos P, d'Arminio Monforte A, Yust I, Bruun JN, Phillips AN, Lundgren JD. Changing patterns of mortality across Europe in patients infected with HIV-1. EuroSIDA Study Group. *Lancet*. 1998;352:1725-1730.

[59] Herberman RB, Nunn ME, Holden HT, Lavrin DH. Natural cytotoxic reactivity of mouse lymphoid cells against syngeneic and allogeneic tumors. II. Characterization of effector cells. *Int J Cancer*. 1975;16:230-239.

[60] Becker S, Kiessling R, Lee N, Klein G. Modulation of sensitivity to natural killer cell lysis after in vitro explantation of a mouse lymphoma. *J Natl Cancer Inst*. 1978;61:1495-1498.

[61] zur Hausen H. Papillomaviruses and cancer: from basic studies to clinical application. *Nat Rev Cancer*. 2002;2:342-350

[62] Heard I, Palefsky JM, Kazatchkine MD. The impact of HIV antiviral therapy on human papillomavirus (HPV) infections and HPV-related diseases. *Antivir Ther*. 2004;9:13-22

[63] Palefsky JM. Cervical human papillomavirus infection and cervical intraepithelial neoplasia in women positive for human immunodeficiency virus in the era of highly active antiretroviral therapy. *Curr Opin Oncol*. 2003;15:382-388

[64] Piketty C, Darragh TM, Heard I, Da Costa M, Bruneval P, Kazatchkine MD, Palefsky JM. High prevalence of anal squamous intraepithelial lesions in HIV-positive men despite the use of highly active antiretroviral therapy. *Sex Transm Dis*. 2004;31:96-99

[65] Stebbing J, Portsmouth S, Fox P, Brock C, Bower M. Multiple human papillomavirus types appear to be a feature of anal not cervical intra-epithelial neoplasia. *Aids*. 2003;17:2401

[66] Fox P, Stebbing J, Portsmouth S, Winston A, Frances N, Nelson M, Gazzard B, Bower M. Lack of response of anal intra-epithelial neoplasia to highly active antiretroviral therapy. *Aids*. 2003;17:279-280

[67] Mbulaiteye SM, Parkin DM, Rabkin CS. Epidemiology of AIDS-related malignancies an international perspective. *Hematol Oncol Clin North Am*. 2003;17:673-696, v.

[68] Mbanya DN, Minkoulou EM, Kaptue LN. HIV-1 infection in adults with haematological malignancies in Yaounde, Cameroon. *West Afr J Med*. 2002;21:183-184.

[69] Dal Maso L, Franceschi S. Epidemiology of non-Hodgkin lymphomas and other haemolymphopoietic neoplasms in people with AIDS. *Lancet Oncol*. 2003;4:110-119.

In: AIDS- Related Opportunistic Infections
Editor: Claudia D. Galanda

ISBN: 978-1-60692-144-9

Chapter IX

Serial Analysis of Gene Expression (SAGE) in African Endemic- and AIDS-Related Kaposi's Sarcoma

Antoinette C. van der Kuyl[1,*], Remco van den Burg[1], Fokla Zorgdrager[1], Celeste Lebbé[2] and Marion Cornelissen[1]

[1] Laboratory of Experimental Virology, Department of Medical Microbiology, Centre of Infection and Immunity Amsterdam (CINIMA), Academic Medical Centre of the University of Amsterdam, Amsterdam, The Netherlands

[2]Department of Dermatology, Centre Hospitalier Universitaire Saint-Louis, 1, Avenue Claude-Vellefaux, Paris, France

Abstract

Kaposi's sarcoma (KS) is subdivided into four epidemiological variants, all of which have in common a similar histopathology and expression of human herpes virus 8 (HHV-8) in the lesions. Two forms are associated with immune suppression, post-transplant KS and AIDS-related KS, while the two others, classic KS and African endemic KS are not. HHV-8 infections are normally benign, with the incidence of HHV-8 infection being much higher than the incidence of KS. The cellular deregulation that leads to the formation of KS lesions is poorly understood, as is the infected cell type. It is also unknown whether gene expression patterns are similar between the epidemiological forms, especially as two forms are not associated with immune dysfunction. To gain insight into the genes expressed in KS lesions, we have generated Serial Analysis of Gene Expression (SAGE) libraries from both AIDS-KS and African endemic KS tissue to analyze mRNA levels in KS. The SAGE libraries were compared with each other and

* Correspondence concerning this article should be addressed to A.C. van der Kuyl, Laboratory of Experimental Virology, Department of Medical Microbiology, Centre of Infection and Immunity Amsterdam (CINIMA), Academic Medical Centre of the University of Amsterdam, Meibergdreef 15, 1105 AZ Amsterdam, The Netherlands.

with libraries in the SAGEmap database. Systematic analysis of the level of gene expression of twelve specific gene families or related genes, including HHV-8 genes, was performed for both endemic KS and AIDS-KS tissue. The results suggested that endemic KS and AIDS-KS have a similar pattern of gene expression, in line with their comparable histopathology.

High or very high expression was found in KS compared with other libraries for psoriasin, HLA-C, complement component 1, keratin 16, galectin 9, plexin D1, CD51, CD31, CCL18, CCL19, CCL21, and many other genes. In general, not the tag counts but rather the tag count ratio of KS versus other libraries gave information about the level of gene expression. Interestingly, a few genes were overexpressed in AIDS-KS compared with endemic KS (e.g. Von Willebrand Factor, D component of complement), while others were overexpressed in endemic KS (e.g. HLA-F, MMP-12, CD74, calgranulin-A).

It has been suggested that iron is an important factor in the establishment of KS. Analysis of iron-related gene expression in KS, however, suggested no clear abnormalities. Relatively high expression was only found for the light polypeptide of ferritin, and heme oxygenase-1, and intermediate expression was seen for the hemoglobin scavenger receptor CD163, compatible with macrophage-related iron-uptake as erythrocytes leak from abnormal vessels in the KS lesions.

In conclusion, the comparison of gene family expression in KS SAGE libraries has provided new insights into the molecular mechanism involved in the pathogenesis of KS.

Keywords: Kaposi'sarcoma, endemic, AIDS, HHV-8, SAGE, gene expression

Introduction

Even though Kaposi's sarcoma (KS) was already described more than a century ago, the disease process at the cellular level is still not completely clear, e.g. whether it is predominantly a hyperplastic or a neoplastic process. Massive neoangiogenesis, extravasation of red blood cells, hemosiderin deposits, whorls of spindle-shaped cells surrounding slit-like spaces, and the presence of a substantial inflammatory infiltrate characterize KS lesions. Progression from patch-, plaque-, to nodular stages is frequent in KS, as is clinical progression from mucocutaneous involvement to visceral disease. The increased incidence of KS in AIDS patients has revived the interest in this otherwise rare disease, and led to the discovery of human herpes virus-8 (HHV-8) replication in the lesions [1]. However, the exact nature of the lesions, as well as the cell type (s) involved, are still the subject of much research and debate (see e.g. [2]). To begin with, the name sarcoma in Kaposi's sarcoma suggests that KS is a tumour. But KS spindle cells do not fulfill criteria for neoplastic cells: aneuploidy is rare, as are chromosomal rearrangements, cells do not grow permissively in culture, and clonality is infrequently observed [3,4,5], and probably confined to the later stages of the disease. Also, lesions may regress spontaneously. Altogether, a picture emerges of KS as an inflammatory systemic disease, where the multiple lesions occurring simultaneously are not metastases, but seeding of progenitor cells, features already noticed by Moritz Kaposi [6]. That KS progenitor cells are present in otherwise healthy, HHV-8$^+$ persons, that can establish lesions in immunosuppressed patients, became clear after analysis of KS cells in transplant-patients [7].

The origin of KS spindle cells, which express both endothelial and macrophage antigens [8] and are the main HHV-8 infected cell in KS lesions, is another matter of debate. The expression profile of HHV-8- infected endothelial cells of different origin have been examined with gene arrays [9,10,11], and correlated with protein expression in KS lesions [10,11]. The results suggest that endothelial cells in lesions resemble lymphatic endothelial cells better than blood vascular endothelial cells [11], but HHV-8 can reprogram blood vascular endothelium towards lymphatic development [10]. Furthermore, the infection of dermal endothelial cells with HHV-8 induces the expression of macrophage-related genes [9]. Possibly, HHV-8 in vivo infects haemangioblasts (a progenitor of both haematopoietic and endothelial cells), and deregulates their normal maturation, accounting for the aberrant co-expression of macrophage, lymphatic- and blood vascular endothelial markers in KS spindle cells. Yet, spindle cells are not the only cells that contribute to the pathology of KS. Infiltrating macrophages and lymphocytes are also implicated in the process, and are likely involved by paracrine mechanisms.

KS is divided into four epidemiological subtypes: classical KS, African endemic KS, post-transplant KS, and AIDS-related KS that are indistinguishable by histopathology. In all forms, lytic replication of HHV-8 can be detected in the lesions. To investigate total gene expression in KS tissue of different epidemiological origin, the SAGE (Serial Analysis of Gene Expression) method was used to obtain an expression profile from pooled nodal KS tissue of four African patients without HIV infection (African endemic KS), and compare it with SAGE libraries from AIDS-related KS [12], and with all other libraries present in the SAGEmap database (www.ncbi.nlm.nih.gov/SAGE/). Totally, twelve gene families or functionally related genes were analyzed for their expression in KS, including HHV-8 genes, and the results were interpreted in relation to the (uncertainties in the) disease process.

Methods

Patient Material

Biopsies were obtained from nodal KS lesions from four HIV-1 negative male African endemic KS patients: two patients were from Zaire, one patient was from Mali, and the fourth patient originated from Cameroon. The presence of HHV-8 DNA in the endemic KS lesions was tested with a nested HHV-8 PCR before generation of the SAGE library [13]. All KS lesions were HHV-8 DNA positive (data not shown). In addition, frozen sections were cut with a microtome, fixed with acetone and stained with antibodies to HHV-8 LANA (ORF73, Advanced Biotechnologies, MD, USA). Spindle cells in all four lesions showed the typical nuclear dot-like LANA staining pattern (not shown). HIV-1 RT PCR confirmed the absence of HIV-1 RNA in the tissues (data not shown).

Serial Analysis of Gene Expression (SAGE)

A SAGE library was constructed from frozen skin biopsies taken from lesions from four African endemic KS patients. The biopsies were cut with a microtome in 10-14 μm sections for RNA isolation. The SAGE library was constructed from the four pooled tissues using the I-SAGE kit™ from Invitrogen (Carlsbad, CA, USA). Sequencing was done with the Bigdye Terminator Cycle Sequencing kit (ABI, Foster City, CA, USA) and an ABI 377 automated sequencer (ABI, Foster City, CA, USA), using M13 forward and M13 reverse primers on colony inserts.

SAGE Library Analysis

Primary analysis of the SAGE library was performed with USAGE version2 [14]. The program performs initial analyses on raw sequence data, e.g. ditag and tag extraction, tag counting, and tag identification. Tags were identified with the SAGEmap database available through NCBI (www.ncbi.nlm.nih.gov/SAGE/), to which USAGE is directly linked. Viral tags were identified with a USAGE viral database created by extracting relevant SAGE tags from all viral cDNA sequences present in the NCBI database. The program USAGE was also used to compare taglists and to do statistical analyses on tag count differences. Additionally, the endemic KS library (referred to as library KSc) was compared with SAGE libraries generated earlier from two AIDS-KS tissues, referred to as libraries KSa and KSb (GEO accession numbers GSM3240 and GSM3241), respectively [12], and with the complete SAGEmap database that contains over 200 SAGE libraries from multiple tissue types, both normal and diseased.

Results

Histological Staining of African Endemic-KS Tissue

All tissues were collected, snap frozen, and stored at -80°C. Histological staining was performed on the frozen tissue. All four African endemic-KS skin biopsies showed a similar histopathological picture of nodular advanced-stage Kaposi's sarcoma with irregular, dense areas of spindle cell proliferations, that were HHV8-LANA positive (not shown). Ziehl-Neelsen, grotcott and PAS staining demonstrated the KS tissues to be negative for mycobacteria and fungi (data not shown).

Description of the SAGE Library

A total of 48,497 tags were analysed in endemic-KS SAGE library: 1453 tags occurred five times or more, 3491 were seen between two and four times, and 11,482 tags occurred only once. The frequency distribution fits with the overall pattern of gene expression in mammalian cells, wherein only a few percent of mRNA species reach high copy numbers whereas most transcripts display low levels [15].

Tags Differentially Expressed between African Endemic KS and AIDS-related KS

Analysis of the three KS libraries from endemic- and AIDS-related KS did not reveal substantial differences in tags or tag numbers expressed. In total, 76 tags were significantly higher expressed in endemic KS than in AIDS-related KS, while 54 tags were significantly higher expressed in both AIDS-KS libraries than in endemic KS. Tags higher expressed in endemic KS included many tags for HLA proteins, including the invariant chains, and immunoglobulins, suggestive of extensive immune dysfunction in AIDS-related KS. African endemic KS is not associated with immunodeficiency [16]. Tags overexpressed in AIDS-KS included those for the interleukin-1 receptor and for Von Willebrand factor (VWF). HIV-1 infection is known to increase IL-1 expression with negative effects on AIDS-related KS [17]. AIDS-KS cells express very high levels of IL-1 [18] and also express the IL-1 receptor [19]. IL-1R antagonists inhibit spindle-cell formation [19]. IL-1 and IL-1R expression in other forms of KS has not been tested, but as no HIV-1 infection is involved there, IL-1 may be more important in the pathology of AIDS-KS.

AIDS-KS patients demonstrate higher VWF plasma levels than classical KS patients do, and stain more intense for VWF in cutaneous lesional biopsies [20]. Our results suggest that VWF levels in endemic KS could also be lower than in AIDS-KS.

Viral Transcripts in the Endemic-KS SAGE Library

Table 1. HHV-8 tag counts in AIDS-related- and endemic-KS SAGE libraries

For comparison tag numbers for each group were normalized to 50,000.

Tag sequence	HHV-8 ID	AIDS-KSa	AIDS-KSb	Endemic-KSc
TCTCCTGTCG	ORF59 and ORF58 mRNA (DNA replication): secondary lytic gene	8	0	4
TTCAAAAACA	T0.7 transcript: primary lytic gene	5	1	1
TTATACTTTT	T1.1 transcript (NUT-1/PAN): primary lytic gene	5	1	6
TTGGGTCCAC	ORF K4.2, or IE-3: secondary lytic gene	3	1	0
CGCGGCGGTG	ORF 18: secondary lytic gene	3	0	2
ATAAAAAAAA	ORF K8.1 mRNA	0	0	1
GAGCTTCTGA	ORF K2 (vIL-6 gene): primary lytic gene	0	0	3
GTAGGTGAGG	ORF 74 (vGCR): primary lytic gene	0	0	2
GCCACTTACG	ORF72 (v-Cyclin)	0	0	1

HHV-8 derived tags were identified with a SAGE tag database created by extracting SAGE tags from all viral cDNA sequences present in the NCBI database, and are compiled in Table 1. Some HHV-8 encoded mRNAs do not contain an *Nla*III site, e.g. v-MIP II (ORF K4), v-MIP I (ORF K6), and v-FLIP (ORF 71), so they go undetected by our SAGE method. An expanded set of HHV-8 derived transcripts was detected in endemic KS compared with AIDS-related KS, including tags for v-IL6 and v-GCR. Interestingly, type III lytic transcripts, involved in virion formation and structure, were not found in any KS library.

S100 Protein Expression in KS

S100 proteins, the largest group of calcium-binding proteins, have been implicated in both inflammation and cancer. Most of them are located in a cluster on chromosome 1q21, suggestive of a common regulatory mechanism, but their individual expression is tissue- and cell-type related. Earlier analysis has shown that some S100 proteins are expressed at high levels in AIDS-related KS [12]. We have analysed the complete S100 mRNA expression in both AIDS-related KS and endemic KS by extracting tags for all known human S100 mRNA's from the UniGene database and determining their counts in our KS SAGE libraries (Table 2). Overall, tags for ten out of 18 known S100 proteins were consistently detected in the KS SAGE libraries. From these ten, S100A7, S100A8, and S100A9 were highly expressed compared with other SAGEmap libraries, while moderate expression was found for S100A2, S100A4, and S100A14. Low-level expression was seen for S100A6, S100A10, S100A11, and S100A16.

High expression of S100A7 is seen in many skin diseases and in invasive breast cancer (for a review, see: [21]). It has been linked to the abnormal epidermal differentiation, inflammation and the cellular infiltration seen in those conditions. Both AIDS-related KS and endemic KS skin lesions show high expression of S100A7 mRNA (Table 2), supporting its role in inflammatory skin disease. The S100 proteins A8, A9 and A12 are phagocytic proinflammatory molecules [22]. High expression of S100A8/A9, as observed in our KS SAGE libraries (Table 2), has been implicated in uncontrolled and harmful inflammation [23]. Unfortunately, S100A12 mRNA cannot be measured by our SAGE analysis, as it lacks an *NlaIII* restriction site.

Several S100 proteins have been implicated in cancer or tumour progression. High expression of S100A4, S100A6 and S100B was associated with specific types of cancer, including melanoma, while significant S100A2 expression was seen in lymphoma [24]. Of these, only S100A6 mRNA was detected at intermediate levels in KS, while expression of the other mRNA's was either low or absent (Table 2). Also, upregulation of S100A16 expression, of which moderate levels are expressed ubiquitously, has been associated with malignant transformation [25]. No such upregulation is detectable in KS (Table 2).

Table 2. S100 protein tag counts in AIDS-related- and endemic-KS SAGE libraries

For comparison tag numbers for each group were normalized to 50,000.

Gene	Tag	AIDS-KSa	AIDS-KSb	Endemic-KSc	Expression level compared with other SAGEmap libraries
S100A2	GATCTTTTGG GATCTCTTGG	0 4	0 1	0 29	Low
S100A4	ATGTGTAACG	3	6	5	Low
S100A6	CCCCCTGGAT	10	37	37	Intermediate
S100A7 (Psoriasin 1)	GAGCAGCGCC	182	19	126	High (KSa, KSc)
S100A8 (Calgranulin A)	TACCTGCAGA	63	22	525	High (KSc)
S100A9 (Calgranulin B)	GTGGCCACGG	149	43	126	High
S100A10 (Calpactin 1)	AGCAGATCAG	32	58	38	Intermediate
S100A11 (Calgizzarin)	CAGGCCCCAC	23	33	45	Intermediate
S100A12 (Calgranulin C)	No tag, mRNA lacks *NlaIII* restriction-site	-	-	-	Expression cannot be measured by SAGE
S100A14	TGGGGAGAGG	9	7	8	Low
S100A15	TTCCCTTATA GAGCGGCGCC	0 1	0 0	0 0	-
S100A16	AGCAGGAGCA	5	12	20	Intermediate-low

No tags were detected in the KS SAGE libraries for: S100A1, S100A3, S100A5, S100A13, S100B (neural), and S100P.

MHC-Related Gene Expression in KS

To escape from cytotoxic T-cell (CTL) surveillance, HHV-8 encodes two proteins, K3 and K5, that downregulate MHC class I expression from infected cell surfaces by targeting the MHC proteins for degradation. In addition, HIV-1 vpu- and nef-proteins have similar functions, albeit by different mechanisms (for a review, see: [26]). To investigate a possible effect upon the mRNA levels of MHC-related proteins in KS, we have tabulated all MHC-related genes for which SAGE tags were available (Table 3). Overall, MHC class I genes are highly expressed in both AIDS-related KS and endemic KS, and their tag counts, including those for the invariant chain beta-2-microglobulin, belong among the highest measured in the SAGEmap database. Tags for HLA-G, which is normally limited to the placental trophoblast, are absent. Tag counts for the B-cell specific HLA-F are very high in endemic KS, but are only moderate in AIDS-related KS. The absence of tags for HLA-C in library AIDS-KSa is possibly due to an undetermined genetic variation (the tissue from which it was generated originated from a patient of Asian descent).

MHC class II expression is much lower in KS (and in the complete SAGEmap database) than is class I expression, and is less consistent among the three libraries (Table 3). Invariant chain (CD74) expression is approximately 10 times higher in endemic KS than in AIDS-related KS. The variable HLA-DQB1 and HLA-DPA1 genes are also overexpressed in endemic KS compared to AIDS-related KS.

Table 3. Tag counts of MHC- related genes in AIDS-related- and endemic-KS SAGE libraries

Gene	MHC class	Tag	AIDS-KSa	AIDS-KSb	Endemic-KSc	Expression level compared with other SAGEmap libraries
HLA-A	I	AGAAAAAAAA GTGCACTGAG AGAACCTTCC	4 114 64	2 130 16	75 144 111	Tag has multiple ID's High (tag could also be HLA-C) High
HLA-B	I	CTGACCTGTG	57	127	157	High
HLA-C	I	GTGCGCTGAG	0	186	32	Very high (KSb), high (KSc)
HLA-E	I	AGGGGCTACC ACCCTTTAAC	0 13	0 7	1 20	High (KSc) High (KSa/KSc)
HLA-F	I	TGCAGCACGA	1	10	79	Very high (KSc)
Beta-2-microglobulin	I	GTTGTGGTTA	262	266	688	Very high (KSc), moderate (KSa, KSb)
HLA-DRB3	II	GTGTGTCTGA ACAGCGCTGA	0 0	0 0	2 3	Moderate (KSc) Moderate-low (KSc)
HLA-DQA1	II	TCCAGTAACA CCTGGGGTAA	0 4	0 0	0 9	Generally: very low expression Moderate (KSa/KSc)
HLA-DQA2	II	GGCATTGTGG GAAGCAATAA	0 1	0 2	0 4	Generally: very low expression Low, unreliable tag
HLA-DQB1	II	ATCCTGAGTT	7	4	57	Moderate (KSa/KSb), high (KSc)
HLA-DQB2	II	ACAAACAAAA	0	1	0	Low
HLA-DPA1	II	TGAAAACTAC	0	1	19	Low (KSa/KSb), moderate (KSc)
HLA-DMA	II	CTGACAGTGA	1	4	3	Moderate
HLA-DMB	II	CCTCTCCAAC	2	0	4	High (KSa/KSc)
CD74	II	GTTCACATTA	51	48	469	Very high (KSc), moderate (KSa, KSb)

For comparison tag numbers for each group were normalized to 50,000.

No tags were detected in the KS SAGE libraries for: HLA-G (class I, very low expression in SAGEmap), HLA-DPB1 (class II, tag TTTTATCATT is unreliable), HLA-DOA (class II), HLA-DOB (class II, low expression in SAGEmap), and HLA-DRA (class II, low expression in SAGEmap).

Complement Component Expression in KS

The complement system, consisting of the classical, alternative and lectin-binding activation pathways, is a major element of the innate immune response. The system is normally tightly regulated, as uncontrolled complement activation causes severe inflammatory damage to the host. HHV-8 encodes a viral homologue of a complement regulator (KCP/ORF 4) that is involved in establishing viral latency by enabling escape from complement-mediated virus clearance [27,28]. This gene is only expressed in infected B-cells

[28], suggesting that complement in possibly not downregulated in KS lesions. In line with this hypothesis high expression of complement component 1 q subcomponent was detected earlier in AIDS-related KS [12].

Table 4. Tag counts of complement components in AIDS-related- and endemic-KS SAGE libraries

Gene	Tag	AIDS -KSa	AIDS -KSb	Endemi c-KSc	Expression level compared with other SAGEmap libraries
Complement component 1, q subcomponent, alpha polypeptide	CTCTAAGAAG	64	16	26	Very high (KSa), high (KSb, KSc)
Complement component 1, q subcomponent, beta polypeptide	GAGGGTGCCA	21	22	7	High (KSa, KSb), Moderate (KSc)
Complement component 1 q subcomponent, gamma-polypeptide	AAATCAATAC	6	11	8	Moderate
Complement component 1, s subcomponent	ACTGAAAGAA	4	5	2	Moderate
Complement component 1, r subcomponent	TTCTGTGCTG	19	50	2	Very high (KSb), high (KSa)
Complement component 1, q subcomponent binding protein	ATAGACATAA	0	1	0	Low
Complement component 1, q subcomponent, receptor 1	CTGATTAGGA	1	0	0	High (KSa)
Complement component 3	GTTGTCTTTG	19	24	7	Moderate (KSa, KSb)
Complement component 4A	AACACAGCCT	6	5	1	Low
Complement component 5, receptor 1	ACTTTAATGA	1	0	4	Moderate (KSc), low (KSa)
Complement component 7	AGTGACTGTG	1	1	0	-
Complement component 8, beta polypeptide	CCTGTGCCAA (unreliable tag)	0	0	1	High (KSc)
D component of complement (adipsin)	GAGGTGGGTG	1	3	0	Very high (KSa, KSb)
Properdin P factor, complement	TCTACACGTG	0	0	1	Moderate (KSc)
Complement S protein (vitronectin)	GCCGGGCCCT	0	1	0	Low (KSb)
B factor, properdin (complement)	GCAGGCCAAG	1	4	0	Low (KSa, KSb)
Complement component 1 inhibitor (SERPING 1)	CTCTCCAAAC	2	3	1	Moderate
Complement component 4, binding protein, beta	ACAATGGAGG	0	0	1	Moderate (KSc)
H factor 1 (complement)	TATGGAGAAT	0	1	0	Low
Membrane cofactor protein (CD46)	CTTTTCAAGA	0	2	2	Low (KSb, KSc)
DAF (CD55)	GGCTTGCTGA	2	1	1	Low

No tags were detected in the KS SAGE libraries for: complement component 1 r subcomponent-like, complement component 2, complement component 3A receptor 1, complement component receptor 2 (CD21), complement component receptor 3 alpha (CD11b), complement component 5, complement component 6, complement component 8 alpha polypeptide, complement component 8 gamma polypeptide, complement component 9 (only expression in liver), complement component 4 binding protein alpha, I factor (complement), complement component 3B/4B, receptor 1 (CD35), and CD59.

Table 5. Iron-related genes expressed in KS SAGE libraries

Gene	Tag	AIDS -KSa	AIDS -KSb	Endemic-KSc	Expression level compared with other SAGEmap libraries
SLC40A1: ferroportin	GAGACTGCAA	6	7	13	Intermediate
FTH1: ferritin, heavy polypeptide	TTGGGGTTTC	106	132	234	Intermediate
ACO1: aconitase 1, soluble	GATAGGTCGG	5	2	2	Low
SLC39A1: solute carrier family 39 (zinc transporter), member 1	CCCAGATGAT	4	1	0	Intermediate
UQCRF: ubiquinol-cytochrome c reductase, Rieske iron-sulfur protein	GGTCACACTA	0	1	5	Low
TF: transferrin	TGTGCTGAAC TATTAGTTAT	0 0	1 0	0 0	Very low
FRDA: Friedreich ataxia, frataxin	AGCTGCTGGC	0	1	0	Low
HEPH: hephaestin, ferroxidase	TTTTAGACAG	0	2	0	Low
TFR2: transferrin receptor 2	GGCCGTGGAG	0	1	0	Low
FTL: ferritin, light polypeptide	CCCTGGGTTC	164	237	210	High
SLC11A1: solute carrier family 11 (proton-coupled divalent metal ion transporters), member 1	CTGGCCAGGC	0	3	3	Moderate (KSb, KSc)
SLC11A2: solute carrier family 11 (proton-coupled divalent metal ion transporters), member 2	AAATAATTGT	0	0	1	Low
HIF1A: hypoxia-inducible factor 1, alpha subunit	TAGATTTCAA	0	0	1	Low
HBA2: hemoglobin, alpha 2	CTTCTTGCCC CCCAACGCGC	0 0	30 123	5 5	Low-intermediate (KSb) High (KSb), low (KSc)
LCN2: lipocalin 2, oncogene 24p3	TGCCCTCAGG	0	0	2	Low
HBB: hemoglobin, beta	GCAAGAAAGT	0	49	7	Low-intermediate (KSb)
LTF: lactoferrin	GCAAAACAAC	1	0	1	Very low, unreliable tag
MYC: v-myc	ATCAAATGCA	0	1	0	Very low
CYP17A1: cytochrome P450, family 17, subfamily A, polypeptide 1	GCCTGGCTGC	1	0	0	High (KSa)
EGLN2 (Egl nine homolog 2 (C. elegans)	GGTGTGGAAG	4	1	10	Intermediate
MFI2: antigen p97, melanotransferrin precursor	GCCAAGACCT ACCATACAAA	0 0	1 0	0 0	High (KSb)
HMOX1: heme oxygenase (decycling) 1	CGTGGGTGGG	276	66	203	High
HMOX2: heme oxygenase (decycling) 2	GGTGACTATC	0	1	0	Intermediate (KSb)
BLVRA: biliverdin reductase A	TTGGGGAAAC	3	1	6	High (KSc), moderate (KSb), low (KSb)
BLVRB: biliverdin reductase B	AGGAGCAAA G	11	3	2	Moderate (KSsa), low (KSb, KSc)
RHCE: rhesus blood group, CcEe antigens	ACAGCAAAGT ACAGCAAAGC	0 0	1 0	0 0	High (KSb)
PRKWNK4: protein kinase, lysine deficient 4	GAGCTTGTGT	0	0	1	Intermediate (KSc)
FTHL17: ferritin, heavy polypeptide-like 17	TTGCCCTTTC	0	0	1	Intermediate (KSc)
CYP2A6: cytochrome P450, family 2, subfamily A, polypeptide 6	AGCTTCCTGC	0	0	3	Intermediate (KSc)
CD163: hemoglobin scavenger receptor	AGTCAGCTGA	1	5	2	Intermediate-high (KSb)

For comparison tag numbers for each group were normalized to 50,000.

No tags were detected in the KS SAGE libraries for: HFE (hemochromatosis), TFRC (transferrin receptor, CD71), ANK1 (ankyrin 1, erythrocyte), ABCB7 (ATP-binding cassette, subfamily B (MDR/TAP), member 7), NFE2 (nuclear factor erythroid-derived 2, 45kDa), HAO1 (hydroxyacid oxidase 1, glycolate oxidase), PRKWNK1 (protein kinase, lysine deficient 1), ABCB6 (ATP-binding cassette, subfamily B (MDR/TAP), member 6), EGLN1 (Egl nine homolog 1 (C. elegans)), PX (hemopexin), HBD (hemoglobin, delta), HBG (hemoglobin, gamma), CA4 (carbonic anhydrase IV), FDX1 (ferredoxin 1), FECH (ferrochelatase), and ALAS2 (aminolevulinate, delta-, synthase 2).

We have analysed complement expression in KS by tabulating all available tags for complement components and their counts in the three KS libraries (Table 4). Indeed, high tag counts for classical pathway complement component 1 subcomponents were seen in both AIDS-related and endemic KS. Of the alternative pathway, for which counts are generally low in the SAGEmap database, only relatively high expression of the D component was seen in AIDS-related KS. Expression of regulators of complement was either low or absent in KS (lower nine tags in Table 4).

Together these results are suggestive of a dysregulated expression of components of complement of at least the classical pathway in KS, with especially high expression of the complement component 1 subcomponents and a low presence of regulators of complement activation. This dysregulation could well contribute to the disease process in KS.

KS and Iron Metabolism

KS lesions are characterized by massive neoangiogenesis of leaky vessels from which erythrocytes extravasate into the surrounding tissue. Large numbers of haemosiderin-laden macrophages and ferritin granules are present in the KS lesions. Also, heme oxygenase-1, the rate-limiting enzyme in the degradation of heme, is highly expressed in KS lesions [12,29], and is induced upon HHV-8 infection of endothelial cells [29]. It has been suggested that iron is a possible co-factor in the pathogenesis of KS [30,31,32], although treatment of KS patients with the iron chelator desferrioxamine resulted in enhancement of symptoms [33,34]. To analyse the role of iron-related gene expression in KS, we have searched the NCBI databases OMIM and UniGene for "iron", which resulted in 45 gene hits other than enzymes containing catalytic iron. The extracted tags and their counts in the KS SAGE libraries are shown in Table 5. A total of 15 of these genes were not expressed in KS at all, while for the other 30 genes expression was generally low compared with other SAGE libraries. Relative high expression was detected for the light (L) polypeptide of ferritin, and for heme oxygenase-1. Consistent (in all three libraries) moderate till high expressed was the heavy (H) polypeptide of ferritin, and the hemoglobin scavenger receptor CD163. The higher expression of the L-polypeptide of ferritin could indicate that ferritin in KS lesions is L-rich, as in iron-storing organs (liver and spleen). L-rich ferritin can bind more iron than H-rich ferritin, which might be beneficial in KS. The hemoglobin scavenger receptor CD163 mediates the endocytosis of hemoglobin:haptoglobin complexes, is expressed by anti-inflammatory macrophages, and induces both IL-10 and heme oxygenase-1 [35]. The latter enzyme is also highly expressed in KS lesions.

Keratins and Keratin-Binding Proteins in KS

Some keratin genes, including constitutive epidermal keratins and keratins involved in hyperproliferation, are highly expressed in AIDS-related KS tissue [12]. To complete the list of keratins expressed in KS, we have analysed the tag counts of keratins and keratin-binding

Table 6. Keratins and keratin-binding proteins expressed in KS SAGE libraries

For comparison tag numbers for each group were normalized to 50,000.

Gene*	Tag	AIDS-KSa	AIDS-KSb	Endemic-KSc	Expression level compared with other SAGEmap libraries
Keratin 2A	CCTCTTTGCA	0	1	2	Moderate (KSb, KSc)
Keratin 5	GCCCCTGCTG	62	102	132	Moderate
Keratin 6A	AAGCACAAG	17	20	57	Moderate (Ksa, KSb), high (KSc)
Keratin 6B	CGAATGTCCT	0	4	34	Moderate (KSc), low (KSb)
Keratin 6E	TCAAGAAGCA	0	0	1	Moderate (KSc)
Keratin 7	CCTGGTCCCA	2	5	0	Low
Keratin 8	CCTCCAGCTA	1	1	0	Low
Keratin 10	GAAAACAAAG	7	20	26	Moderate (KSa), high (KSb, KSc)
Keratin 14	GATGTGCACG	35	50	28	Moderately high
Keratin 15	TAATAAAGAA	0	0	4	Low, tag has second reliable ID
Keratin 16	CAGCTGTCCC	12	12	28	High
Keratin 17	CTTCCTTGCC	22	20	97	Moderate (KSa, KSb), high (KSc)
Keratin 18	CAAACCATCC	2	6	4	Low
Keratin 19	GACATCAAGT	0	1	0	Low
Keratin 23	AGACCAATGA	0	1	0	Moderate (KSb)
Envoplakin	GTGATGGGCT	1	2	1	Moderate
Desmoplakin	ACAGCGGCAA	26	31	28	High
Bullous phemphigoid antigen 1, 230/240kDa	TTCTGGTATT TGAGGTTTTC TGAGAATAAT GTAAATATGG	0 1 0 0	1 0 0 0	1 0 0 1	Low Low - Low
Periplakin	AAAATAAACC	1	0	2	Moderate (KSa, KSc)
Plectin	TTCCACTAAC	3	3	2	Low
Vimentin	TCCAAATCGA	0	12	129	Moderate (KSb), high (KSc)
Desmin	CCCCGGCCAC	1	9	0	Moderate (KSa), high (KSb)

*Hair keratins have not been included. No tags were detected in the KS SAGE libraries for: keratin 1, keratin 1B, keratin 3, keratin 4, keratin 5B, keratin 6L, keratin 9, keratin 12 (only expressed in eye), keratin 13, keratin 20 (expressed in intestinal epithelium), keratin 24, keratin 25A, keratin 25C, keratin 25D, nor for any keratin-associated protein, or for any UniGene entry with the description “similar to keratin x”.

proteins in both AIDS-related KS and endemic KS (Table 6). Expression of some cytokeratins, e.g. keratins 5, 10, 14, and 18, was consistently found in all three libraries. As in the earlier analysis [12], keratins 6A and 16 were also detected at moderate to high levels in AIDS-KS and endemic KS (Table 6). These keratin genes are rapidly induced in the epidermis upon wounding or inflammation. Cytokeratin 17, expressed by basal “stem” cells in complex epithelia, was also consistently detected in the three KS libraries. Of the proteins interacting with keratin, desmoplakin was highly expressed in all three libraries, while periplakin, vimentin and desmin were only expressed in two out of three libraries. High expression for vimentin was seen in endemic KS with moderate expression in AIDS-KSb, while desmin, which is mainly expressed in muscle, was highly expressed in AIDS-KSb. Vimentin, an intermediate filament protein which was formerly thought to only participate in stabilization of the cytoplasmic architecture, is also abundantly secreted by activated macrophages [36], suggesting it has a function in the immune response. In addition, binding of the heavy chain of IgG to cytoskeletal vimentin can activate the classical pathway of the complement cascade *in vitro* [37].

Galectin Expression in KS

Of the 10 known human galectins and galectin-like proteins for which a reliable tag is available, galectins 1, 3, 7, and 9 are expressed in all three KS SAGE libraries, while low expression of galectin 2 is seen in endemic KS (Table 7). Galectins display a vast array of functions, both intra- and extra-cellular (for a review see: [38]). Amongst others, galectins are involved in inflammation (for a review see: [39]), regulation of immune responses (for a review see: [40]), and fulfil yet unclear roles in cancer processes (for a review see: [41]). Especially galectins 1 and 3 are speculated to play an important role in inflammatory-induced tissue destruction. Both are mainly expressed by epithelium, endothelium and activated tissue macrophages, but have generally opposite effects in inflammation. Galectin 1 is a negative regulator of the immune response, whilst galectin 3 is a pro-inflammatory molecule, which enhances cell adhesion and prevents T-cell apoptosis. Galectins 7, expressed only in stratified epithelia, and galectin 9 also have multiple regulatory roles in inflammation and immune processes [42]. Galectin 9 is expressed in many tissues, and in endothelial cells after stimulation with interferon-gamma [42].

So, the final effects of galectin expression in KS are unclear, but it is likely that changing levels of galectins exert a profound influence upon the disease process.

Table 7. Galectin expression in KS SAGE libraries

For comparison tag numbers for each group were normalized to 50,000.

Gene*	Tag	AIDS-KSa	AIDS-KSb	Endemic-KSc	Expression level compared with other SAGEmap libraries
Galectin 1	TTTTTTGTAA	0	0	1	Low
	GTACCCGTAC	0	0	0	-
	GCCCCCAATA	65	75	157	Moderate (KSa, KSb) high (KSc)
Galectin 2	TCCTCTTTCA	0	0	2	Moderate (KSc)
Galectin 3	TTCACTGTGA	16	31	27	Moderate
Galectin 7	TAAACCTGCT	28	77	20	Moderate
Galectin 9	CTCAGTCCCC	3	1	1	High

* Galectin 5 is only found in rat, galectin 6 is only found in mouse, OvGal11 is only found in sheep/cow. No tags were detected in the KS SAGE libraries for: galectin 4, galectin 8, galectin 12, galectin 13, and HSPC159.

Semaphorin, Plexin and Neuropilin Expression in KS

Semaphorins are a family of highly conserved signalling molecules with diverse functions, including cell migration, immune response, angiogenesis, and tumour growth and metastasis (for a review see: [43]). Two types of semaphorin receptor have been identified: the plexins and the neuropilins. Currently, the presence of any of these molecules in KS has not been investigated. Therefore, we have tabulated all known tags for semaphorins, plexins and neuropilins, and their counts in the three KS SAGE libraries (Table 8). As can be seen from this table, at least 5 semaphorin tags are consistently expressed in KS. However, three of these tags do not have a unique ID, a severe drawback of the SAGE method, so that their expression cannot unequivocally be attributed to a specific gene. Leaving out these three tags, we can conclude that at least Sema3C and Sema6B are expressed in KS, while Sema3D is expressed in endemic KS, and Sema3F in AIDS-related KS. SEMA3 proteins are involved in endothelial cell migration and angiogenesis through the regulation of integrin function [44]. Unfortunately, the tag derived from SEMA3A mRNA, the best studied of these proteins, is absent from the KS libraries, and is not expressed in the complete SAGEmap database. Possibly, the mRNA for Sema3A deposited in the database is not correct, or otherwise the mRNA could be expressed at very limited occasions. Tags for the semaphorin receptors are either low or absent, or have a double ID (as for neuropilin 2). Surprisingly, the only one of these tags highly expressed in both AIDS-related and endemic KS is the one for the atypical plexin D1, which is known to be involved in embryonic angiogenesis in mice, and is expressed by endothelial cells in vascular endothelium [45]. Our results suggest that plexin D1 is also involved in the development of blood vessels in Kaposi's sarcoma. It has been speculated that as plexins of the B and C subfamilies bind semaphorin classes 4 and 7, respectively, and the neuropilins are the receptors for class 3 semaphorins, plexins of the A and D subfamilies could be the receptor for the other semaphorin subclasses [46]. In mice, however, SEMA3E was shown to be the ligand for plexin D1 [47].

Table 8. Semaphorin, plexin and neuropilin expression in KS SAGE libraries

For comparison tag numbers for each group were normalized to 50,000.

Gene	Tag	AIDS -KSa	AIDS-KSb	Endemic -KSc	Expression level compared with other SAGEmap libraries
Semaphorin 3C	TTGAATTCCC	1	1	5	Low
Semaphorin 3D	ACTGTTCTAT	0	0	3	High (KSc)
Semaphorin 3E	AGGTCAGGAG	22	24	10	Tag has at least 15 reliable ID's
Semaphorin 3F	GATGCGAGGA	3	2	0	High (KSa, KSb)
Semaphorin 4A	CAGGGATCTG	1	0	1	Moderate
Semaphorin 4C	TGTTTGTGTG	4	1	6	Moderate-high, tag has a second reliable ID
Semaphorin 4D	ATAGGATTTG	0	0	1	Moderate (KSc), tag has a second reliable ID
Semaphorin 4F	GCTCTAGGCT	0	1	0	Moderate (KSb)

Table 8. Continued

Gene	Tag	AIDS -KSa	AIDS-KSb	Endemic -KSc	Expression level compared with other SAGEmap libraries
Semaphorin 6B	CCACGTGGCT	10	5	2	High (KSa), moderate (KSb, KSc)
Semaphorin 6C	GTGACTGCCA	9	13	19	Tag has a second reliable ID
Semaphorin 6D	TAAAGTCAAA	1	0	0	Low
	CACATACATA	0	0	0	-
Plexin A1	ATTGTGCTAG	1	0	0	-
	TTCGACTTCC	0	0	0	-
Plexin A4*	TGGGAGACGG	0	0	0	-
	GAATAAAATA	0	0	3	Low, tag has a second reliable ID
Plexin B1	GTGAGGGCTA	0	1	0	Low
Plexin B2	CCCTAGGTTG	0	1	0	Low
Plexin D1	GGGGCTGGAG	29	27	37	Very high
Plexin domain containing 1 (TEM7)	CATTTTTATC	1	0	0	Moderate (KSa)
Neuropilin 1	TTTTGTACCA	0	1	0	Low
Neuropilin 2	TGTGTGTGTG	6	3	1	Tag has 7 other reliable ID's
	CTGGGGATGC	0	0	0	-
	AATGACAAGA	0	0	0	-
ESDN, endothelial and smooth muscle cell-derived neuropilin-like protein	TACTGTAGTC	0	0	1	Low

* No mRNA is known for plexin A3.

No tags were detected in the KS SAGE libraries for: semaphorin 3A (note: tag AGTAACTTTC has never been seen in any SAGEmap database), semaphorin 3B, semaphorin 4B, semaphorin 4G, semaphorin 5A, semaphorin 5B, semaphorin 6A, semaphorin 7A, LOC56920 (semaphorin sem 2), plexin A2, plexin B3, plexin C1, plexin domain containing 2, likely ortholog of mouse plexin 3, NETO1 (neuropilin and tolloid-like 1), and NETO2 (neuropilin and tolloid-like 2).

Adhesion Molecule Expression in KS SAGE Libraries

Massive leukocyte infiltrates are a hallmark of inflammation and of (early) KS. Several molecules have been implicated in leukocyte adhesion, e.g. selectins, integrins, and members of the immunoglobulin superfamily (e.g. ICAM, VCAM). To study mRNA expression of these adhesion-related molecules in KS, all tags available for entries of these families in the UniGene database were retrieved from SAGEmap (Table 9).

Selectins (L-, P, and E-selectin) were not consistently expressed in the three KS SAGE libraries. However, tag counts for selectins are low in the SAGEmap database, suggesting that expression of these genes cannot accurately be measured using SAGE.

Table 9. Adhesion molecules expressed in KS SAGE libraries

Gene	Tag	AIDS-KSa	AIDS-KSb	Endemic-KSc	Expression level compared with other SAGEmap libraries
L-selectin	CAATTTTGCA	0	0	3	High (KSc)
P-selectin (CD62)	TCACCGTGGA	3	0	2	High (KSa, KSc)
Integrin, alpha 3	GTACTGTAGC	2	1	1	Low
Integrin, alpha 5	ATGGCAACAG	13	16	1	Moderate (KSa, KSb), tag has second reliable ID
Integrin, alpha 6	ATTAGAAATT	1	0	0	Low
Integrin, alpha 7	GGGTAGGGTG	0	3	0	Moderate
Integrin, alpha D	CCACTGCACT	418	350	89	High, tag has multiple reliable IDs
Integrin, alpha E (CD103)	GAGCTGTTGG	6	4	2	High (Ksa, KSb), moderate (KSc)
Integrin, alpha L (CD11a)	TATTTATCCA	2	0	1	Moderate
Integrin, alpha V (CD51)	TAACTTGTGA	20	7	35	High
Integrin, alpha X (CD11c)	CACAAAAAGA	0	0	4	High (KSc)
Integrin, beta 1 (CD29)	TGAAGTTATA CAGCCCAGAA ACAGAAGGGA	3 0 1	3 0 2	6 0 1	Low Low Low
Integrin, beta 2 (CD18)	GAGACTTGAG	0	2	1	Moderate (KSb, KSc)
Integrin, beta 4	AAGGGGGCAA	0	7	0	Moderate (KSb)
Integrin, beta 5	CCAGGCTGCG	5	10	2	High (KSb), moderate (KSa, KSc)
ICAM 1 (CD54)	GTTCACTGCA	0	3	0	Moderate (KSb)
ICAM 2	GCCACCACCA	3	3	3	Moderately high
ICAM 3	TTAGGGAGGA	2	0	0	Moderate (KSa)
VCAM 1	GTACGGAGAT	5	0	2	High (Ksa), moderate (KSc)
PECAM 1 (CD31)	CTGAAGGCTG	10	11	14	Very high
JAM 3	GGAACCAGGT	1	4	2	High (KSb), moderate (KSa, KSc)
CEACAM 1	TCTGAATTAT	1	0	0	Low
ESAM	AAATATGTGT	0	2	0	Moderate (KSb)
DSCAM	ACTGGACAGC	2	1	0	Moderate (KSa, KSb)
CEECAM 1	TTGCCCAGCA	5	20	2	High (KSb), moderate (KSa, KSc)
NRCAM	AAAGGGTCAC	1	0	0	Low
MCAM (CD146)	GGGATTAAAG	0	0	7	High (KSc)
Vascular adhesion protein 1 (AOC3)	TGACTGTATT	1	3	1	High (KSb), moderate (KSa, KSc)
ADRM1	AGCCTGGACT	10	7	1	High (KSa, KSb), low (KSc)
ASAM	GTGCCAGGCA	0	3	1	Moderate (KSb), low (KSc)
CD44	AAGATTGGGG	0	1	3	Low
Ninjurin 1	AATGAACAAT	3	1	7	Moderate (KSc), low (KSa, KSb)
E-cadherin	TGTGGGTGCT	4	2	1	Low
H-cadherin	CACACACACA	3	2	1	Moderate
OB-cadherin	TAAGAAAATG	0	0	2	Moderate (KSc)
P-cadherin	TACGGTGGCG	0	0	2	Moderate (KSc)
VE-cadherin	ACAAGTACTG	21	8	14	High
M-cadherin	CAAAAAAAAA	1	3	33	Tag has many reliable IDs
Vitronectin	GCCGGGCCCT	0	1	0	Low (KSb)
Fibronectin	GTGTCAGATA ATCTTGTTAC	0 8	1 18	0 17	Low (KSb) Moderate
VWF	TTCTGCTCTT	21	28	6	High (KSa, KSb), moderate (KSc)

For comparison tag numbers for each group were normalized to 50,000.

No tags were detected in the KS SAGE libraries for: selectin E, integrin alpha 1, integrin alpha 2, integrin alpha 2b, integrin alpha 4, integrin alpha 8, integrin alpha 9, integrin alpha 10, integrin alpha 11, integrin alpha M (CD11b), integrin beta 6, integrin beta 7, integrin beta 8, ICAM 4, ICAM 5, NCAM 1, NCAM 2, L1CAM, ALCAM, DSCAML1, AMICA, JAM 1, JAM 2, SPAM 1, MADCAM 1, PUNC, CEACAM 3, CEACAM 4, CEACAM 5, CEACAM 6, CEACAM 7, CEACAM 8, OPCML, neurofascin, CD226, N-cadherin, KSP-cadherin, R-cadherin, and all type 2 cadherins.

Integrins that are consistently expressed in KS are integrin α3, integrin αV, integrin β1, and integrin β5. The highest expression was measured for integrin αV and integrin β5. Immunohistochemistry has shown that integrins αV, α5, and β1 are expressed by both spindle cells and by the endothelium in KS lesions, while integrins α3 and β3 were only expressed by the endothelium [48]. Integrin β5 was not studied. Tags derived from integrin α5 and αD mRNA's do not have an unique ID, rendering them useless for this analysis. Integrin αV, *in vivo* part of the vitronectin receptors (integrin αVβ3 and integrin αVβ5), has been described as a negative regulator of angiogenesis, although it is often highly expressed on angiogenic blood vessels [49]. Antibodies directed against integrin αVβ3 were found to target KS tumour cells and inhibit tumour growth in a nude mouse model of KS [50]. Surprisingly, proangiogenic integrins, e.g. integrin α5β1 and its ligand fibronectin, are expressed at much lower levels in KS than the angiogenesis inhibiting integrin αVβ5. Integrin α3β1, which is expressed in KS at low levels, can function as a cellular receptor for HHV-8 [51].

Adhesion molecules of the immunoglobulin superfamily that were always expressed in the KS SAGE libraries were ICAM2 (which is constitutively expressed by endothelial cells), PECAM 1 (CD31, a well-known marker for KS lesions), JAM3 (junctional adhesion molecule 3, involved in leukocyte transmigration through the endothelial barrier), and CEECAM1 (cerebral endothelial cell adhesion molecule 1). Other adhesion molecules consistently expressed are AOC3, also named vascular adhesion protein 1, an endothelial sialoglycoprotein whose cell surface expression is induced under inflammatory conditions, and ADRM1, a gamma-interferon-inducible gene. Of the cadherins, calcium-binding proteins that mediate cell-cell interactions, only VE-cadherin is highly expressed in KS, while H-cadherin and E-cadherin are moderately or lowly expressed, respectively. Downregulation of E-cadherin has been associated with cancer progression (for a review see: [52]). Expression of E-cadherin in KS is lower than in normal skin (not shown), suggestive of downregulation. In most cancer types, however, loss of E-cadherin expression is accompanied by a gain in mesenchymal cadherin expression (N-cadherin and OB-cadherin, known as the "cadherin-switch"), which is not evident in KS (Table 9). In skin tumours, downregulation of H-cadherin is associated with increased invasiveness as well.

Table 9 also lists a few ligands for adhesion molecules, of which especially Von Willebrand factor (VWF) is highly expressed in AIDS-KS, and somewhat lower in endemic KS. VWF is mainly synthesized by endothelial cells, can bind to the αVβ3 and αVβ5 integrins, and has been reported to be elevated in plasma from $HIV\text{-}1^+$ patients and patients with AIDS-related KS (for a review, see: [53]), and to a lower extent in patients with classic KS [20]. Generally, increased expression of VWF is an indication for endothelial damage and activation.

Matricellular and Basement Membrane Protein Expression in KS SAGE Libraries

Members of the matricellular protein family are functionally related, minor constituents of the extracellular matrix (ECM) that appear only shortly upon specific developmental or pathological events. They include thrombospondins, tenascins, CCN family members, osteopontin, and osteonectin (for a review, see: [54]). Matricellular proteins are involved in T-cell maturation and ECM remodelling. In all three KS libraries highly expressed are osteonectin and thrombospondin 3 (Table 10). Lower expression was found for hevin, CCN1, CCN2, and WISP-2. Cartilage oligomeric matrix protein (COMP) is highly expressed in a single AIDS-KS library, but is found at only a moderate level in the other two libraries. Inconsistent expression was found for osteopontin, thrombospondin 1 and 2, tenascin C, tenascin XB, and NOV. Surprisingly, tenascin C that is highly induced early in inflammatory processes, and at the invasion borders of malignant tumours [55], is barely detectable in our KS libraries.

Of the CCN family of matricellular proteins, CCN1 (CYR61), and CCN2 (connective tissue growth factor), both produced by endothelial cells, are important regulators of angiogenesis [56], and both are expressed in KS. So, matricellular protein family members are widely present in KS, in line with the extensive ECM remodelling observed in KS lesions.

Of the basement membrane proteins, high-level mRNA expression in all three KS libraries was detected for type IV collagens alpha 1 and alpha 2, and laminins alpha 4 and beta 1 (Table 10). Consistent, but lower expression was seen for alpha 5 laminin (Table 10). Laminin alpha 4 has been implicated in angiogenesis, as it is necessary for the development of microvessels [57]. Fibulins are notably expressed in blood vessels, but are also found as part of basement membranes (for reviews, see: [58,59]). Fibulin 1C is expressed in all three KS libraries, while fibulins 1D, 2, and 5 are found in only one or two libraries. Fibulin 5 has been shown to promote endothelial cell adhesion, and fulfil a role in vascular development and remodelling [60].

Table 10. Matricellular and basement membrane protein mRNA

expression in KS SAGE libraries

Gene	Tag	AIDS -KSa	AIDS -KSb	Endemic-KSc	Expression level compared with other SAGEmap libraries
Osteopontin	AATAGAAATT	1	0	0	Low (KSa)
Osteonectin	ATGTGAAGAG	112	130	365	Very high (KSc), high (KSa, KSb)
Thrombospondin 1	AGGTCTTCAA	0	4	1	Low (KSb, KSc)
Thrombospondin 2	AAAAAAAAAA	6	5	110	Tag has multiple reliable IDs
Thrombospondin 3	CGAGGGGGGC	3	4	2	High
COMP	CGGGGTGGCC	2	54	4	Very high (KSb), moderate (KSa, KSc)
Hevin	TGCACTTCAA	25	65	13	High (KSb), moderate (KSa, KSb)
Tenascin C	AAGCTGTATA	1	3	0	Moderate (KSb), low (KSa)
Tenascin XB	AGCTACCACA	0	3	1	Moderate (KSb, KSc)
CYR61 (CCN1)	AGTGTCTGTG	4	9	2	Moderate (KSa, KSb), low (KSc)
CTGF (CCN2)	TTTGCACCTT	26	14	14	Moderate
NOV	TATCTGGTTT	0	1	0	Moderate (KSb)
WISP-2	CACACGGGCG	1	13	3	High (KSb), moderate (KSc), low (KSa)
Collagen, type IV, alpha 1	GACCGCAGGA	56	179	137	Very high (KSb, KSc), high (KSa)
Collagen, type IV, alpha 2	TTCTCCCAAA	6	3	6	High (KSa, KSc), moderate (KSb)

Table 10. Continued

Gene	Tag	AIDS-KSa	AIDS-KSb	Endemic-KSc	Expression level compared with other SAGEmap libraries
Laminin, alpha 1	TGCAACAAAT	0	1	0	Moderate (KSb)
Laminin, alpha 2	TACATAGAAT	0	4	3	High (KSb, KSc)
Laminin, alpha 4	ACAGAGCACA	9	17	15	Very high (KSb, KSc), high (KSa)
Laminin, alpha 5	ACTCGCTCTG	2	5	2	Moderate (KSb), low (KSa, KSc)
Laminin, beta 1	CTTGTAACAG	6	11	7	Very high (KSb), high (KSa, KSc)
Laminin, beta 2	TCTGCCTATG	6	1	0	High (KSa), low (KSb)
Laminin, beta 3	CCATTGAAAC	0	1	1	Low
Laminin, gamma 2	GTGAAACCCT GGGGCACTTG	20 0	59 0	50 0	Tag has many reliable IDs
Laminin, gamma 3	CATAAACGGG	0	1	3	High (KSc), moderate (KSb)
Perlecan	CCACCCTCAC	1	0	1	Low
Nidogen 1	ACCTCACCCC	1	0	1	High (KSa, KSc)
Nidogen 2	TGATCAATAT	0	2	1	High (KSb, KSc)
Fibulin 1C	CAGCTGGCCA	6	19	6	High (KSb), moderate (KSa, KSc)
Fibulin 1D	ACAGAATGCC	6	12	0	High (KSb), moderate (KSa)
Fibulin 2	TACATTATAT	0	3	0	High (KSb)
Fibulin 4	AGCTACCGGG	1	4	0	Moderate (KSb), low (KSa)
Fibulin 5	CTATGTTCTG	0	3	1	High (KSb), moderate (KSc)

For comparison tag numbers for each group were normalized to 50,000.

No tags were detected in the KS SAGE libraries for: thrombospondin 4, tenascin N, tenascin R, WISP-1, WISP-3, collagen type IV alpha 3, collagen type IV alpha 4, collagen type IV alpha 5, collagen type IV alpha 6, agrin, laminin alpha 3, laminin beta 2, laminin gamma 1, fibulin 1A, fibulin 1B, fibulin 3, and fibulin 6.

MMP and TIMP Expression in KS SAGE Libraries

Matrix metalloproteinases and their inhibitors play an important role in angiogenesis and degradation of the extracellular matrix, and are involved in tissue remodelling and invasion. MMP-2, MMP-9, MMP-12, and MMP-19, and sometimes MMP-1, are expressed in KS lesions [61]. MMP-12, exclusively produced by CD68+ macrophages, was mainly detected in advanced nodular KS lesions, which was also true for MMP-9 [61]. Clinical trials in KS patients with an MMP inhibitor were promising [62], confirming the importance of MMP expression in disease progression.

Table 11 shows tags for MMP's and their inhibitors (TIMP's: tissue inhibitors of metalloproteinases) detected in KS. Consistent expression was seen for MMP-1, MMP-2, MMP-15, MMP-25, TIMP-1, and TIMP-3. MMP-18 (=MMP-19) and MMP-12 expression was only seen in endemic KS. MMP-28, which is increased in basal keratinocytes during tissue repair [63], was detected in two out of three KS libraries. Besides MMPs, another extracellular matrix degrading enzyme, cathepsin B, is also highly expressed in KS (91 tags in KSa, 66 tags in KSb, and 35 tags in KSc).

TIMP's have multiple activities besides inhibition of MMP's (for a review, see: [64]). The high expression of TIMP-1, an inducible TIMP, has not been described before in KS. TIMP-1 has been shown to have cell-growth promoting and anti-apoptotic activities. However, in cancer, overexpression of TIMP-1 and TIMP-2 is beneficial, while downregulation is associated with increased invasiveness [64].

Table 11. MMP and TIMP expression in KS SAGE libraries

Gene	Tag	AIDS-KSa	AIDS-KSb	Endemic-KSc	Expression level compared with other SAGEmap libraries
MMP-1	TGCAGTCACT	9	3	10	High (KSa, KSc), moderate (KSb)
MMP-2	GGAAATGTCA	14	38	50	High (KSb, KSc), moderate (KSa)
MMP-7	AACTTGGCCA	0	1	0	Unreliable tag
MMP-9	TAAATCCCCA	1	0	1	Moderate (KSa, KSc)
MMP-11	CAGGAGACCC	0	1	3	Moderate (KSb, KSc)
MMP-12	CTCTGTAAGT	0	0	11	Very high (KSc)
MMP-14	GTACCGGGGA	0	1	1	High (KSb, KSc)
MMP-15	GCCCTGAGCG	1	1	1	Moderate
MMP-17	ACCTCTCCCT	2	0	6	High (KSc), moderate (KSa)
MMP-18 (=MMP-19)	TTCATAAAAA GAAGACAGTG	0 0	0 0	2 0	Moderate (KSc) -
MMP-25	TATGAGGAGG AGTTTGGCCA AGGACAGAAG	1 0 1	1 0 0	1 0 2	Moderate - Low (Ksa), moderate (KSc)
MMP-28	GATGGGGATG	1	0	1	Moderate (KSa, KSc)
TIMP-1	GAGAGTGTCT	14	48	10	Very high (KSb), moderate (KSa, KSc)
TIMP-2	AATAAAACAC	1	0	0	Tag has second reliable ID
TIMP-3	TTATTTATGA	1	1	1	Low

For comparison tag numbers for each group were normalized to 50,000.
No tags were detected in the KS SAGE libraries for: MMP-3, MMP-8 (=MMP-27), MMP-10, MMP-13, MMP-16, MMP-20, MMP-21, MMP-23B, MMP-24, MMP-26, and TIMP-4.

Chemokine Expression in KS SAGE Libraries

Chemokines (for a review, see: [65]) play an important role in the establishment of Kaposi's sarcoma, as many different cell types are attracted to the lesions. Both IL-8 (CXCL8) and GRO-alpha (CXCL1) are known growth factors for KS, and are involved in KS angiogenesis [66,67]. To survey the possible expression of other chemokine genes in KS, we have collected tags for all classes of human chemokines, and tabulated their counts in the three KS SAGE libraries (Table 12). Several chemokines were inconsistently expressed between the three libraries, including CXCL8 (IL-8), which was virtually absent from the AIDS-related KS libraries, but was moderately expressed in endemic KS (Table 12). Highly expressed in all three libraries were tags for CCL18, CCL19, CCL21, CXCL14, and CXCL16. In addition, CCL27 was highly expressed in AIDS-related KS.

CC chemokines are subdivided into four groups plus the structurally unique CCL27. Only members of the pro-inflammatory (CCL3, CCL4, CCL18) and homeostatic subgroups (CCL19, CCL21), but none of the allergenic and developmental subgroups are found in KS. Some consider CCL19 and CCL20 to be pro-inflammatory chemokines [68]. CCL18 is expressed at a low level by dendritic cells, and at a high level by alternatively activated macrophages [69]. This subset of macrophages is mainly found in healing wounds and in chronic inflammation, and is highly angiogenic [70].

Table 12. Chemokine expression in KS SAGE libraries

For comparison tag numbers for each group were normalized to 50,000.

Gene	Tag	AIDS-KSa	AIDS-KSb	Endemic-KSc	Expression level compared with other SAGEmap libraries
CCL2*	GTACTAGTGT	1	0	3	Low
CCL3	GCACCAAAGC	1	0	12	Low
CCL4	GATAACACAT	0	0	6	Moderate (KSc)
CCL5 (Rantes)	AAAAATCGGC	0	1	2	Low
CCL8	GATCATCAAG	0	0	1	Moderate (KSc)
CCL13	AAGGGATGCT	1	1	0	High, rare tag
CCL17	GGCACAAAGG	0	0	1	Moderate (KSc)
CCL18	GATCAATCAG	5	23	13	Very high (KSb), high (KSa, KSc)
CCL19	GCCCTGCTAC	1	2	1	Very high (KSb), high (KSa, KSc)
CCL21	AGAGGAGGCA	6	5	8	Very high
CCL22	GACAAGGATG	0	0	0	-
	AACGGGGCCC	0	0	1	Moderate (KSc)
CCL26	GACCCGCTGG	1	0	0	Moderate (KSa)
CCL27	GGACTCTGCC	1	5	0	High (KSb), rare tag
XCL2	AATAAAATTA	0	0	1	Tag has a second reliable ID
CXCL2**	TTGAAGCTTT	0	1	0	Low
CXCL3	ATAATAAAAG	0	0	5	Low
CXCL6	TTGGTTTTTG	0	0	3	Moderate (KSc)
CXCL8 (IL-8)	TGGAAGCACT	1	0	22	Moderate (KSc), low (KSa)
CXCL9	CATACACTCT	2	2	4	Moderate
CXCL12	TAGAAAATTT	0	0	1	Moderate (KSc)
	GTATAAACGT	2	0	0	Moderate (KSa)
CXCL14	CAGGTTTCAT	14	24	26	High
CXCL16	CCTGGCCCTA	2	1	2	High
SCYE1	AGCAACAGTG	1	6	1	High (KSb), low (KSa, KSc)

*CCL = chemokine (C-C motif) ligand; **CXCL= chemokine (C-X-C motif) ligand

No tags were detected in the KS SAGE libraries for: CCL1, CCL7, CCL11, CCL15, CCL16, CCL20, CCL23, CCL24, CCL25, CCL28, XCL1, CXCL1, CXCL4, CXCL5, CXCL7, CXCL10, CXCL11, CXCL13.

CCL19 and CCL21 are two chemokines using CCR7 as a receptor; both are downregulated by IL-10, and both play a role in T-cell adhesion. CCL21 is overexpressed in endothelial cells of T-cell mediated skin diseases, while CCL19 expression in disease is less clear, and was only seen in a single case of atopic dermatitis [71]. CCL27 is constitutively expressed by basal keratinocytes and also attracts T-cells, but was not overexpressed in several human autoimmune skin diseases [71].

Of the CXC chemokines, members of the ELR-motif (+) group (CXCL3, CXCL6, and CXCL8 are detected in KS) are much lower expressed than members of the ELR-motif negative group (CXCL9, CXCL14 and CXCL16 are found in KS), which are chemotactic for monocytes (CXCL9, CXCL14) and T-cells (CXCL9, CXCL16). CXC chemokines are involved in the mediation of inflammation and the angiogenesis balance (for a review, see: [72]). Interestingly, CXC chemokines with angiogenic properties (CXCL2, CXCL3, CXCL6, CXCL8, and CXCL12) are, albeit weakly, more often expressed in KS than angiostatic chemokines (CXCL9, Table 12), suggesting that an imbalance of CXC chemokine mediated angionesis, which finally leads to transformation and tumour progression, contributes significantly to the disease process in KS.

Tags for chemokine receptors were investigated, but repeatedly found to be negative. Only two single tags for CCR5 and CCR10, respectively, were detected (result not shown). In general, tags representing receptor mRNA's are difficult to detect using SAGE, suggesting that these mRNA's are present in lower concentrations than mRNA's coding for other types of proteins.

Conclusion

The novel approach of analyzing gene family expression in nodal Kaposi's sarcoma lesions as measured by the SAGE method contributes to the common perception of the disease as an uncontrolled inflammatory, rather than a primary neoplastic process. Of the S100 protein mRNA's, the pro-inflammatory subset (S100A7, S100A8, S100A9) involved in unrestrained and harmful inflammation was highly expressed, rather than the subset implicated in cancer or tumour progression (e.g. S100A2, S100A4, S100A6, S100B). In addition, high levels of pro-inflammatory chemokine mRNA's were found in the tissues, together with high and aberrant expression of complement components, another cause of severe inflammatory damage. Keratin 6A and 16 mRNA, both induced by wounding and inflammation, were prominently present in KS tissue, as was TIMP-1 mRNA, which is believed to be beneficial and is associated with reduced invasiveness in cancer.

Analysis of iron-related gene expression in KS was not suggestive of any pecularity despite the suggested role of iron in the disease. Significant expression was detected only for the light polypeptide of ferritin, heme oxygenase-1, and the hemoglobin scavenger receptor CD163, compatible with macrophage-related iron-uptake as erythrocytes leak from the abnormal vessels found in KS.

As expected, genes involved in ECM remodelling and angiogenesis were also prominently expressed in KS, as were adhesion molecules. In further disagreement with a neoplastic process is the absence of the cadherin switch (loss of E-cadherin expression accompanied by a gain in N-cadherin or OB-cadherin expression) in KS lesions. Plexin D1 mRNA, originally implicated in embryonic angiogenesis, is highly expressed in KS, suggestive of a function in the development of blood vessels in KS. Probably, it also plays a role in neoangiogenesis in other non-embryonic tissues.

Furthermore, the results suggested that endemic KS and AIDS-related KS have a similar pattern of gene expression, in line with their comparable histopathology. Very few genes, mainly MHC-related, but also Von Willebrand factor (VWF), D component of complement, MMP-12, and calgranulin-A, are differentially expressed between the two forms of KS.

References

[1] Chang, Y., Cesarman, E., Pessin, M. S., Lee, F., Culpepper, J., Knowles, D. M., and Moore, P. S. (1994). Identification of herpesvirus-like DNA sequences in AIDS-associated Kaposi's sarcoma. *Science, 266*, 1865-1869.

[2] Perez, A., Sanchez, J. L., and Almodovar, P. I. (2003). Kaposi's sarcoma is not a neoplasm let alone a sarcoma. *Int. J Dermatol., 42*, 844-845.

[3] Delabesse, E., Oksenhendler, E., Lebbe, C., Verola, O., Varet, B., and Turhan, A. G. (1997). Molecular analysis of clonality in Kaposi's sarcoma. *J Clin Pathol., 50*, 664-668.

[4] Rabkin, C. S., Janz, S., Lash, A., Coleman, A. E., Musaba, E., Liotta, L., Biggar, R. J., and Zhuang, Z. (1997). Monoclonal origin of multicentric Kaposi's sarcoma lesions. *N Engl J Med, 336*, 988-993.

[5] Gill, P. S., Tsai, Y. C., Rao, A. P., Spruck, C. H., III, Zheng, T., Harrington, W. A., Jr., Cheung, T., Nathwani, B., and Jones, P. A. (1998). Evidence for multiclonality in multicentric Kaposi's sarcoma. *Proc Natl Acad Sci U S A, 95*, 8257-8261.

[6] Kaposi, M. (1872). Idiopathic multiple pigmented sarcoma of the skin. *Arch. Dermatol. Syphilol, 4*, 265-273.

[7] Barozzi, P., Luppi, M., Facchetti, F., Mecucci, C., Alu, M., Sarid, R., Rasini, V., Ravazzini, L., Rossi, E., Festa, S., Crescenzi, B., Wolf, D. G., Schulz, T. F., and Torelli, G. (2003). Post-transplant Kaposi sarcoma originates from the seeding of donor-derived progenitors. *Nat. Med, 9*, 554-561.

[8] Uccini, S., Ruco, L. P., Monardo, F., Stoppacciaro, A., Dejana, E., La Parola, I. L., Cerimele, D., and Baroni, C. D. (1994). Co-expression of endothelial cell and macrophage antigens in Kaposi's sarcoma cells. *J. Pathol., 173*, 23-31.

[9] Poole, L. J., Yu, Y., Kim, P. S., Zheng, Q. Z., Pevsner, J., and Hayward, G. S. (2002). Altered Patterns of Cellular Gene Expression in Dermal Microvascular Endothelial Cells Infected with Kaposi's Sarcoma-Associated Herpesvirus. *J. Virol., 76*, 3395-3420.

[10] Hong, Y. K., Foreman, K., Shin, J. W., Hirakawa, S., Curry, C. L., Sage, D. R., Libermann, T., Dezube, B. J., Fingeroth, J. D., and Detmar, M. (2004). Lymphatic reprogramming of blood vascular endothelium by Kaposi sarcoma-associated herpesvirus. *Nat. Genet., 36*, 683-685.

[11] Wang, H. W., Trotter, M. W., Lagos, D., Bourboulia, D., Henderson, S., Makinen, T., Elliman, S., Flanagan, A. M., Alitalo, K., and Boshoff, C. (2004). Kaposi sarcoma herpesvirus-induced cellular reprogramming contributes to the lymphatic endothelial gene expression in Kaposi sarcoma. *Nat. Genet., 36*, 687-693.

[12] Cornelissen, M., van der Kuyl, A. C., van den Burg R., Zorgdrager, F., van Noesel, C. J., and Goudsmit, J. (2003). Gene expression profile of AIDS-related Kaposi's sarcoma. *BMC Cancer, 3*, 7-

[13] Goudsmit, J., Renwick, N., Dukers, N. H. T. M., Coutinho, R. A., Heisterkamp, S., Bakker, M., Schulz, T. F., Cornelissen, M., and Weverling, G. J. (2000). Human herpesvirus 8 infections in the Amsterdam Cohort Studies (1984- 1997): Analysis seroconversions to ORF65 and ORF73. *Proceedings of the National Academy of Sciences of the United States of America, 97*, 4838-4843.

[14] van Kampen, A. H., van Schaik, B. D., Pauws, E., Michiels, E. M., Ruijter, J. M., Caron, H. N., Versteeg, R., Heisterkamp, S. H., Leunissen, J. A., Baas, F., and van der Mee, M. (2000). USAGE: a web-based approach towards the analysis of SAGE data. *Bioinformatics., 16*, 899-905.

[15] Hastie, N. D. and Bishop, J. O. (1976). The expression of three abundance classes of messenger RNA in mouse tissues. *Cell, 9*, 761-774.

[16] Kestens, L., Melbye, M., Biggar, R. J., Stevens, W. J., Piot, P., De Muynck, A., Taelman, H., De Feyter, M., Paluku, L., and Gigase, P. L. (1985). Endemic African Kaposi's sarcoma is not associated with immunodeficiency. *Int. J Cancer, 36*, 49-54.

[17] Corley, P. A. (1997). Induction of interleukin-1 and glucocorticoid hormones by HIV promotes viral replication and links human chromosome 2 to AIDS pathogenesis: genetic mechanisms and therapeutic implications. *Med Hypotheses, 48*, 415-421.

[18] Ensoli, B., Nakamura, S., Salahuddin, S. Z., Biberfeld, P., Larsson, L., Beaver, B., Wong-Staal, F., and Gallo, R. C. (1989). AIDS-Kaposi's sarcoma-derived cells express cytokines with autocrine and paracrine growth effects. *Science, 243*, 223-226.

[19] Louie, S., Cai, J., Law, R., Lin, G., Lunardi-Iskandar, Y., Jung, B., Masood, R., and Gill, P. (1995). Effects of interleukin-1 and interleukin-1 receptor antagonist in AIDS-Kaposi's sarcoma. *J Acquir Immune Defic Syndr. Hum Retrovirol., 8*, 455-460.

[20] Janier, M., Flageul, B., Drouet, L., Scrobohaci, M. L., Villette, J. M., Palangie, A., and Cottenot, F. (1988). Cutaneous and plasma values of von Willebrand factor in AIDS: a marker of endothelial stimulation? *J Invest Dermatol., 90*, 703-707.

[21] Watson, P. H., Leygue, E. R., and Murphy, L. C. (1998). Psoriasin (S100A7). *Int. J Biochem Cell Biol, 30*, 567-571.

[22] Roth, J., Vogl, T., Sorg, C., and Sunderkotter, C. (2003). Phagocyte-specific S100 proteins: a novel group of proinflammatory molecules. *Trends Immunol, 24*, 155-158.

[23] Sampson, B., Fagerhol, M. K., Sunderkotter, C., Golden, B. E., Richmond, P., Klein, N., Kovar, I. Z., Beattie, J. H., Wolska-Kusnierz, B., Saito, Y., and Roth, J. (2002). Hyperzincaemia and hypercalprotectinaemia: a new disorder of zinc metabolism. *Lancet, 360*, 1742-1745.

[24] Hsieh, H. L., Schafer, B. W., Sasaki, N., and Heizmann, C. W. (2003). Expression analysis of S100 proteins and RAGE in human tumors using tissue microarrays. *Biochem Biophys. Res Commun., 307*, 375-381.

[25] Marenholz, I. and Heizmann, C. W. (2004). S100A16, a ubiquitously expressed EF-hand protein which is up-regulated in tumors. *Biochem Biophys. Res Commun., 313*, 237-244.

[26] Fruh, K., Bartee, E., Gouveia, K., and Mansouri, M. (2002). Immune evasion by a novel family of viral PHD/LAP-finger proteins of gamma-2 herpesviruses and poxviruses. *Virus Res, 88*, 55-69.

[27] Spiller, O. B., Blackbourn, D. J., Mark, L., Proctor, D. G., and Blom, A. M. (2003). Functional activity of the complement regulator encoded by Kaposi's sarcoma-associated herpesvirus. *J Biol Chem, 278*, 9283-9289.

[28] Spiller, O. B., Robinson, M., O'Donnell, E., Milligan, S., Morgan, B. P., Davison, A. J., and Blackbourn, D. J. (2003). Complement regulation by Kaposi's sarcoma-associated herpesvirus ORF4 protein. *J Virol, 77*, 592-599.

[29] McAllister, S. C., Hansen, S. G., Ruhl, R. A., Raggo, C. M., DeFilippis, V. R., Greenspan, D., Fruh, K., and Moses, A. V. (2004). Kaposi sarcoma-associated herpesvirus (KSHV) induces heme oxygenase-1 expression and activity in KSHV-infected endothelial cells. *Blood, 103*, 3465-3473.

[30] Simonart, T., Noel, J. C., Andrei, G., Parent, D., Van Vooren, J. P., Hermans, P., Lunardi-Yskandar, Y., Lambert, C., Dieye, T., Farber, C. M., Liesnard, C., Snoeck, R., Heenen, M., and Boelaert, J. R. (1998). Iron as a potential co-factor in the pathogenesis of Kaposi's sarcoma? *Int. J Cancer, 78*, 720-726.

[31] Ziegler, J. L., Simonart, T., and Snoeck, R. (2001). Kaposi's sarcoma, oncogenic viruses, and iron. *J Clin Virol, 20*, 127-130.

[32] Simonart, T. (2004). Iron: a target for the management of Kaposi's sarcoma? *BMC Cancer, 4*, 1-

[33] Simonart, T., Boelaert, J. R., Andrei, G., van den Oord, J. J., Degraef, C., Hermans, P., Noel, J. C., Van Vooren, J. P., Heenen, M., De Clercq, E., and Snoeck, R. (2002). Desferrioxamine enhances AIDS-associated Kaposi's sarcoma tumor development in a xenograft model. *Int. J Cancer, 100*, 140-143.

[34] Simonart, T., Boelaert, J. R., and Van Vooren, J. P. (2002). Enhancement of classic Kaposi's sarcoma growth after intralesional injections of desferrioxamine. *Dermatology, 204*, 290-292.

[35] Philippidis, P., Mason, J. C., Evans, B. J., Nadra, I., Taylor, K. M., Haskard, D. O., and Landis, R. C. (2004). Hemoglobin scavenger receptor CD163 mediates interleukin-10 release and heme oxygenase-1 synthesis: antiinflammatory monocyte-macrophage responses in vitro, in resolving skin blisters in vivo, and after cardiopulmonary bypass surgery. *Circ. Res, 94*, 119-126.

[36] Mor-Vaknin, N., Punturieri, A., Sitwala, K., and Markovitz, D. M. (2003). Vimentin is secreted by activated macrophages. *Nat. Cell Biol, 5*, 59-63.

[37] Hansson, G. K., Lagerstedt, E., Bengtsson, A., and Heideman, M. (1987). IgG binding to cytoskeletal intermediate filaments activates the complement cascade. *Exp Cell Res, 170*, 338-350.

[38] Leffler, H., Carlsson, S., Hedlund, M., Qian, Y., and Poirier, F. (2004). Introduction to galectins. *Glycoconj. J*, 19, 433-440.

[39] Almkvist, J. and Karlsson, A. (2004). Galectins as inflammatory mediators. *Glycoconj. J, 19*, 575-581.

[40] Rabinovich, G. A., Toscano, M. A., Ilarregui, J. M., and Rubinstein, N. (2004). Shedding light on the immunomodulatory properties of galectins: novel regulators of innate and adaptive immune responses. *Glycoconj. J, 19*, 565-573.

[41] van den, B. F., Califice, S., and Castronovo, V. (2004). Expression of galectins in cancer: a critical review. *Glycoconj. J, 19*, 537-542.

[42] Hirashima, M., Kashio, Y., Nishi, N., Yamauchi, A., Imaizumi, T. A., Kageshita, T., Saita, N., and Nakamura, T. (2004). Galectin-9 in physiological and pathological conditions. *Glycoconj. J, 19*, 593-600.

[43] Tamagnone, L. and Comoglio, P. M. (2004). To move or not to move? Semaphorin signalling in cell migration. *EMBO Rep., 5*, 356-361.

[44] Serini, G., Valdembri, D., Zanivan, S., Morterra, G., Burkhardt, C., Caccavari, F., Zammataro, L., Primo, L., Tamagnone, L., Logan, M., Tessier-Lavigne, M., Taniguchi, M., Puschel, A. W., and Bussolino, F. (2003). Class 3 semaphorins control vascular morphogenesis by inhibiting integrin function. *Nature, 424*, 391-397.

[45] van der Zwaag B., Hellemons, A. J., Leenders, W. P., Burbach, J. P., Brunner, H. G., Padberg, G. W., and Van Bokhoven, H. (2002). PLEXIN-D1, a novel plexin family member, is expressed in vascular endothelium and the central nervous system during mouse embryogenesis. *Dev. Dyn., 225*, 336-343.

[46] Tamagnone, L., Artigiani, S., Chen, H., He, Z., Ming, G. I., Song, H., Chedotal, A., Winberg, M. L., Goodman, C. S., Poo, M., Tessier-Lavigne, M., and Comoglio, P. M. (1999). Plexins are a large family of receptors for transmembrane, secreted, and GPI-anchored semaphorins in vertebrates. *Cell, 99*, 71-80.

[47] Gu, C., Yoshida, Y., Livet, J., Reimert, D. V., Mann, F., Merte, J., Henderson, C. E., Jessell, T. M., Kolodkin, A. L., and Ginty, D. D. (2005). Semaphorin 3E and plexin-D1 control vascular pattern independently of neuropilins. *Science, 307*, 265-268.

[48] Kaaya, E. E., Castanos-Velez, E., Amir, H., Lema, L., Luande, J., Kitinya, J., Patarroyo, M., and Biberfeld, P. (1996). Expression of adhesion molecules in endemic and epidemic Kaposi's sarcoma. *Histopathology, 29*, 337-346.

[49] Hynes, R. O. (2002). A reevaluation of integrins as regulators of angiogenesis. *Nat. Med, 8*, 918-921.

[50] Rader, C., Popkov, M., Neves, J. A., and Barbas, C. F., III (2002). Integrin alpha(v)beta3 targeted therapy for Kaposi's sarcoma with an in vitro evolved antibody. *FASEB J, 16*, 2000-2002.

[51] Akula, S. M., Pramod, N. P., Wang, F. Z., and Chandran, B. (2002). Integrin alpha3beta1 (CD 49c/29) is a cellular receptor for Kaposi's sarcoma-associated herpesvirus (KSHV/HHV-8) entry into the target cells. *Cell, 108*, 407-419.

[52] Cavallaro, U. and Christofori, G. (2004). Cell adhesion and signalling by cadherins and Ig-CAMs in cancer. *Nat. Rev. Cancer, 4*, 118-132.

[53] de Gaetano, D. K., Rabagliati, R., Iacoviello, L., and Cauda, R. (2004). HIV infection, HAART, and endothelial adhesion molecules: current perspectives. *Lancet Infect. Dis., 4*, 213-222.

[54] Kuznetsova, S. A. and Roberts, D. D. (2004). Functional regulation of T lymphocytes by modulatory extracellular matrix proteins. *Int. J Biochem Cell Biol, 36*, 1126-1134.

[55] Chiquet-Ehrismann, R. and Chiquet, M. (2003). Tenascins: regulation and putative functions during pathological stress. *J Pathol., 200*, 488-499.

[56] Brigstock, D. R. (2002). Regulation of angiogenesis and endothelial cell function by connective tissue growth factor (CTGF) and cysteine-rich 61 (CYR61). *Angiogenesis., 5*, 153-165.

[57] Thyboll, J., Kortesmaa, J., Cao, R., Soininen, R., Wang, L., Iivanainen, A., Sorokin, L., Risling, M., Cao, Y., and Tryggvason, K. (2002). Deletion of the laminin alpha4 chain leads to impaired microvessel maturation. *Mol Cell Biol, 22,* 1194-1202.

[58] Argraves, W. S., Greene, L. M., Cooley, M. A., and Gallagher, W. M. (2003). Fibulins: physiological and disease perspectives. *EMBO Rep., 4*, 1127-1131.

[59] Timpl, R., Sasaki, T., Kostka, G., and Chu, M. L. (2003). Fibulins: a versatile family of extracellular matrix proteins. *Nat. Rev. Mol Cell Biol, 4*, 479-489.

[60] Nakamura, T., Ruiz-Lozano, P., Lindner, V., Yabe, D., Taniwaki, M., Furukawa, Y., Kobuke, K., Tashiro, K., Lu, Z., Andon, N. L., Schaub, R., Matsumori, A., Sasayama, S., Chien, K. R., and Honjo, T. (1999). DANCE, a novel secreted RGD protein expressed in developing, atherosclerotic, and balloon-injured arteries. *J Biol Chem, 274*, 22476-22483.

[61] Impola, U., Cuccuru, M. A., Masala, M. V., Jeskanen, L., Cottoni, F., and Saarialho-Kere, U. (2003). Preliminary communication: matrix metalloproteinases in Kaposi's sarcoma. *Br. J Dermatol., 149*, 905-907.

[62] Cianfrocca, M., Cooley, T. P., Lee, J. Y., Rudek, M. A., Scadden, D. T., Ratner, L., Pluda, J. M., Figg, W. D., Krown, S. E., and Dezube, B. J. (2002). Matrix metalloproteinase inhibitor COL-3 in the treatment of AIDS-related Kaposi's sarcoma: a phase I AIDS malignancy consortium study. *J Clin Oncol., 20*, 153-159.

[63] Lohi, J., Wilson, C. L., Roby, J. D., and Parks, W. C. (2001). Epilysin, a novel human matrix metalloproteinase (MMP-28) expressed in testis and keratinocytes and in response to injury. *J Biol Chem, 276*, 10134-10144.

[64] Lambert, E., Dasse, E., Haye, B., and Petitfrere, E. (2004). TIMPs as multifacial proteins. *Crit Rev. Oncol. Hematol., 49*, 187-198.

[65] Laing, K. J. and Secombes, C. J. (2004). Chemokines. *Dev. Comp Immunol, 28*, 443-460.

[66] Masood, R., Cai, J., Tulpule, A., Zheng, T., Hamilton, A., Sharma, S., Espina, B. M., Smith, D. L., and Gill, P. S. (2001). Interleukin 8 is an autocrine growth factor and a surrogate marker for Kaposi's sarcoma. *Clin Cancer Res, 7*, 2693-2702.

[67] Lane, B. R., Liu, J., Bock, P. J., Schols, D., Coffey, M. J., Strieter, R. M., Polverini, P. J., and Markovitz, D. M. (2002). Interleukin-8 and growth-regulated oncogene alpha mediate angiogenesis in Kaposi's sarcoma. *J Virol, 76*, 11570-11583.

[68] Rossi, D. L., Vicari, A. P., Franz-Bacon, K., McClanahan, T. K., and Zlotnik, A. (1997). Identification through bioinformatics of two new macrophage proinflammatory human chemokines: MIP-3alpha and MIP-3beta. *J Immunol, 158*, 1033-1036.

[69] Kodelja, V., Muller, C., Politz, O., Hakij, N., Orfanos, C. E., and Goerdt, S. (1998). Alternative macrophage activation-associated CC-chemokine-1, a novel structural homologue of macrophage inflammatory protein-1 alpha with a Th2-associated expression pattern. *J Immunol, 160*, 1411-1418.

[70] Kodelja, V., Muller, C., Tenorio, S., Schebesch, C., Orfanos, C. E., and Goerdt, S. (1997). Differences in angiogenic potential of classically vs alternatively activated macrophages. *Immunobiology, 197*, 478-493.

[71] Christopherson, K. W., Hood, A. F., Travers, J. B., Ramsey, H., and Hromas, R. A. (2003). Endothelial induction of the T-cell chemokine CCL21 in T-cell autoimmune diseases. *Blood, 101*, 801-806.

[72] Romagnani, P., Lasagni, L., Annunziato, F., Serio, M., and Romagnani, S. (2004). CXC chemokines: the regulatory link between inflammation and angiogenesis. *Trends Immunol, 25*, 201-209.

In: AIDS- Related Opportunistic Infections
Editor: Claudia D. Galanda
ISBN: 978-1-60692-144-9

Chapter X

Informal Caregiving to Children with HIV/AIDS in Togo: Measures and Concepts

Ami R. Moore
University of North Texas, Denton, Texas, USA

In Africa, it was very common that older family members make important health decisions when young members are sick (Seeley, Kajura, Bachengama, Okongo, Wagner, & Mulder, 1993; Foster 2000). Traditionally, the extended family and clan had been the backbone of the African family system as they had provided help and support to its members whenever needed, especially in times of crises (Foster, 2000). However, because of the unprecedented demands and needs of people living with HIV/AIDS, these institutions may not be able to meet these challenges.

Additionally, because of modernization and individualism prevalent in urban areas, the roles of the extended family in times of need may be weakened (Foster & Williamson, 2000). In fact, AIDS is an exorbitant disease, and currently, most Africans cannot afford effective antiviral therapies. Some families have spent their life savings on loved ones with AIDS but have not seen any improvement in the health of the sick (Moore & Henry, 2005; Family Health International, 2001; UNICEF, 2002). Also, stigma associated with HIV/AIDS has made it difficult for family members to cope with the disease and openly talk about their loved ones who are either HIV positive or have AIDS. Consequently, extended family members or clans may be reluctant to help because of fear of being stigmatized or the inability to care for a sick family or provide assistance because of poverty.

In general, caregiving has a negative impact on the health and well-being of caregivers. Caregiving to people living with AIDS is a stressful activity (Turner & Pearlin, 1989; Pearlin, Aneshensel, & LeBlanc, 1997) that can lead to anxiety and depression (Folkman et al., 199; LeBlanc et al., 1997; Land & Hudson, 2002). Furthermore, caregiving to children with HIV/AIDS is believed to be extraordinarily challenging because when a child is affected usually one parent or both are affected as well (Bettoli-Vaughan et al, 1998). Thus, caring for a child with AIDS can threaten the family unit (Lesar & Maldonato, 1997) by creating additional medical, psychosomatic, and financial strains on the family (Lesar et al, 1995). Living with AIDS affects the family unit as a whole. It changes behaviors of infected children and challenges their physical and mental abilities (Lesar & Maldonato, 1997).

Caregivers of children living with AIDS face many demands on their families' limited resources, both from the children as well as from other infected family members. This only adds to the burden of stress that the caregivers may already be experiencing. However, studies have indicated that effective coping strategies may reduce the level of stress and anxiety among caregivers (McCubbin & Thompson, 1987; Graffi & Minnes, 1989). Furthermore, a few studies report that caregiving has some positive influences on caregivers. For instance, Atkins & Amenta (1991) and Carlisle (2000) found that caregivers obtained benefits and rewards in the process of caring for a person with HIV/AIDS.

The study proposes to examine informal caregiving to children with HIV or AIDS in Togo in order to generate empirical indicators that will be used to develop caregiving measures. Informal caregiving has become an important outlet for people living with AIDS since AIDS is a chronic disease that eventually incapacitates its victims. Moreover, the health care system is poorly developed in Africa (Merson & Rosenfield, 2000), with scarce resources for people with AIDS. Thus, the plight of family members and friends who are caretakers of a loved one with AIDS is compounded.

Researchers have developed instruments to measure the level of stress and anxiety among people giving care to loved ones or close relatives afflicted with chronic and debilitating illnesses; for example the Hopkins Symptom Checklist (Derogatis, Lipman, Rickles, Uhlenhuth, & Covi, 1974); the CES-D measure (Radloff, 1977) and measures of stress by Pearlin, et al. (1990; 1997). Unfortunately, these measures of caregiving experiences have all been developed in the western societies which are economically and culturally different from African societies. Because these measures tend to be culture specific (Aranda & Knight, 1997; Horowitz & Reinhard, 1995), they cannot adequately assess the experiences of informal caregivers in Africa where the effects of HIV/AIDS has been the most severe. Transporting measures from non-African settings may not translate the concepts and experiences of the caregivers in ways that are intelligible and meaningful to African caregivers. Thus, developing instruments to measure caregivers to children with HIV/AIDS is necessary to make intervention programs efficacious. This study attempts to develop an instrument that will measure caregiving experiences of people caring for children with HIV or AIDS in Togo.

Setting

Togo is located in the western coast of Africa. With an estimated population of 6.1 million inhabitants, Togo's primary economic activity is subsistence agriculture (Wikipedia, 2007). A significant percent of the Togolese population was living below the national poverty line: 32.3% in 2002 (UNDP, 2006). An estimated prevalence rate of HIV among adults aged 15 to 49 is 3.2 % with 88,000 AIDS orphans in the beginning of 2007 (UNESCO, 2007). It is noteworthy to report that this prevalence rate has declined from a high of 6% in 2000 (UNAIDS/WHO, 2000). However, the impact of HIV/AIDS in Togo is enormous and especially deleterious among the poor who seem to be the most affected by this epidemic (Moore & Williamson, 2003; Moore & Henry, 2005).

Methods

Participants, Procedure and Analysis

Subjects were convenience-sampled from HIV/AIDS centers in Lomé, Togo. Because of the sensitive nature of the study, we asked the directors at three centers that provide services to people with HIV/AIDS and their families to recruit for the study primary caregivers of children aged 0 to 15 who was HIV positive or had AIDS. We had established working relations with these centers since 2001. It is important to note that 'Unite de Recherche Demographique[2]' in Lomé, Togo--a demographic institute--helped with the study. They provided a demographer statistician, an expert in social and demographic research, who assisted the author with the study.

We explained the study protocol to the directors who selected five of their employees who had at least a Bachelor's degree in Social Sciences to help with the study. The five employees were trained by the author for two days. As part of their training, they also watched the author conduct the first 10 qualitative interviews and later the first 10 surveys. In order to maintain conformity, regular meetings were held to discuss the interviews. To be included, a participant had to be a current primary caregiver and had used the centers' services in the past.

First, through in-depth interviews, the caregiving experiences of 30 caregivers were assessed in July, 2006. Caregivers were asked to give a detailed description of all the things they did from dawn to dusk to the seropositive child. They were also asked to describe ways they managed caregiving demands; for example, what they did specifically when they had ups and downs. They were asked to list all the people they disclosed the serostatus of the child to and the reason(s) for disclosure. They were also asked to list all the family members and others that provided any kind of support and specify what the person did.

Interviews were in French or Ewe (one of the native languages in Togo). They were tape-recorded. They lasted on average about 60 minutes. Tapes were transcribed verbatim. Second, the author and the statistician demographer analyzed the transcripts independently. Quality assurance in the form of inter-coder reliability was enhanced by meetings in which interview content was discussed and conceptual themes debated. Recurrent themes and phrases were classified and grouped into categories. The data were reduced by consensus to key conceptual themes and phrases such as disclosure, coping, impact of antiretroviral drugs (ARVs), etc.

---

[2] Unité de Recherche Démographique is one of the respected research institutes in Togo. It collects data for national and international institutions such as Demographic and Health Surveys (DHS) data for Macro International Inc.

The following section briefly describes the main findings of the qualitative study from which the measures were derived. Caregivers carefully selected people to whom they disclosed the serostatus of the child they were caring for because they feared discrimination and stigma upon disclosure. Most of them did not have any support from family and friends. Family and friends were even at times unaware of the serostatus of the child. Caregivers relied heavily on their faith to overcome the daily challenges of caring for a child with HIV/AIDS. They had substantial financial difficulties meeting the needs of the child they were caring for. For instance, they were for the most part unable to provide nutritious foods to the child. Caring for a child with HIV/AIDS is a taxing activity that affects other activities of the caregivers. For example, most of the caregivers had either stopped their income generating activities or changed them in order to have time to care for the child.

Also, because of the advanced age and the health status of some caregivers, they felt that they should not be caring for a child. Yet, all of the caregivers reported gratitude for having antiretroviral drugs available at a very nominal price, although at times they were financially unable to buy them. Caregivers took extra care for the child because they did not want either to expose the child to other infections or expose others to HIV. Caregivers used different means to cope with the challenges of caring for a child with HIV/AIDS. Some prayed more, others listened more to music.

From the conceptual themes and phrases, we created questions that reflected the caregiving experiences. Whenever possible, we tried to retain verbatim phrases for the questions. It is important to note that, originally, there were 66 items created. However, during the several meetings that we had, the items were reduced to 50 because some did not fit the concepts. These questions were structured following the principal topics gathered from the qualitative study. For instance, from the theme 'disclosure', two categories of questions were created. One depicted caregivers' disclosure of the child's serostatus to family members and the other depicted caregivers' disclosure of the child's serostatus to people they felt can provide them some help. These questions went through a series of pretests and revisions. A set of Likert-style frequency descriptors was used for all response options (4—completely agree; 3—agree; 2—somewhat agree; 1—disagree). The questions were subsequently administered to 207 caregivers from September to December, 2006 in Lomé, the capital city of Togo and the surrounding towns. Because of missing cases, only 201 surveys were analyzed.

Findings

Table 1 presents the descriptive statistics of the caregivers and the children. It can be noted that caregivers were mainly females (about 73%). They were on average 41.66 years and had on average 8.62 years of education. The majority of the caregivers were caring for their nephews or nieces. Most of the caregivers were seronegative (44%). They mostly identified themselves as catholic (about 47%). Over half of the children had lost their biological parents. Most of the children were on ARVs (80%). The ones who were not on therapy were either too young or had a high CD4 count.

The 11 dimensions that describe informal caregiving experiences of children with HIV/AIDS in Togo are: disclosure, expression of faith, financial difficulties, family support, impact of caregiving demands on other activities, personal and social norms, impact of antiretroviral drugs, supplemental efforts made for the child, coping with stress of caregiving, positive comparision, and profound meaning of child's serostatus. Table 2 describes the measures and the reliability (alpha) values. Internal consistency—Cronbach's α for the scales vary from 0.43 (disclosure to families) to 0.91 (supplemental effort). Overall, the scales are relatively quite reliable. Two thirds of the Chronbach's α values are greater than 0.60.

Table 1. Descriptive statistics of caregivers and children caring for

Gender	Female	72.60
	Male	27.40
Marital Status	Married	43.30
	Cohabiting	4.50
	Single	11.90
	Divorce/separated	14.40
	Widowed	25.90
Religion	Catholicism	47.30
	Protestantism	13.40
	Other Christian religion	29.40
	Islam	4.50
	Traditional religion	2.50
	Other	2.10
	None	1.00
Serostatus of caregivers	Positive	32.80
	Negative	43.80
	Don't know	23.40

Table 1. Descriptive statistics of caregivers and children caring for (Continued)

Caregiver's relation to child	Parent	23.40
	Aunt/uncle	39.30
	Grandparent	25.90
	Brother/sister	4.00
	Other	7.40
Status of biological parents of the child		
Father	Deceased	51.70
	Ill	7.00
	Abandoned child	14.40
	Living with child	14.90
	Other	12.40
Mother	Deceased	53.20
	Ill	20.90
	Abandoned child	3.00
	Living with child	17.40
	Other	5.50
Gender of child	Female	54.70
	Male	45.30
Child attending school	Yes	70.10
	No	29.90
Average age caregivers (years)	41.66	
Average years of education	8.62	
Average age children	7.00	
Average monthly expenses	27,601.27 CFA ($1=500)	

Table 2. Constructs and reliability (alpha) of each scale

A. Disclosure

These are some propositions about people with whom you shared the child's positive serostatus.

Which of the propositions best describes your situation? Please answer any one of the statements.

I. Family member **(alpha = 0.43)**

a. Disclose serostatus of child to my family members (2.34).

b. Disclose serostatus of child to members of other family (1.73).

c. Disclose serostatus of child to child's siblings (1.43).

II. Provider of help **(alpha = 0.63)**

a. Disclose child's serostatus to people who can financially help me (2.01).

b. Disclose child's serostatus to people who can emotionally help me (1.78).

c. Disclose child's serostatus to people who can spiritually help me (1.91).

d. Disclose child's serostatus to people who can medically help me (3.70).

B. Expression of faith (0.80)

People who care for children with HIV/AIDS are at times tired of the caregiving demands and resort to other activities to boost themselves up. In what way(s) would you say you have done the following? Please answer each of the statements below by selecting the ones that best describes your case.

a. I go to church (mosque) when I'm tired with caregiving demands (2.72).

b. I pray more when caregiving demands get to me (3.37).

c. I sing Christian (religious) songs when caregiving demands become heavier (2.88).

Table 2: Constructs and reliability (alpha) of each scale (Continued)

B. Expression of faith (0.80)

People who care for children with HIV/AIDS are at times tired of the caregiving demands and resort to other activities to boost themselves up. In what way(s) would you say you have done the following? Please answer each of the statements below by selecting the ones that best describes your case.

d. I listen more to Christian (religious) songs when caregiving demands become difficult (2.91).

e. I ask people to pray for me when caregiving demands become heavier (2.15).

Response categories: (4) Very often; (3) Often; (2) Rarely; (1) Never.

C. Financial difficulties (0.88)

a. I have financial difficulty to feed the child (3.03).

b. I have financial difficulty to provide clothing for the child (3.31).

c. I have financial difficulty to provide leisure for the child (take the child out to the movies, beach, etc.) (3.32).

d. I have financial difficulty to provide sweet treats (candy, ice cream, cake, cookies, etc.) for the child (3.16).

Response categories: (4) Very often; (3) Often; (2) Rarely; (1) Never.

D. Family support (0.59)

Oftentimes, our family members provide different forms of support when we have difficulty, for instance when we are giving care to an ill person. However, we may be at times disappointed by the inaction of our family members. Please in what way(s) have you felt the following from family members?

a. Your brothers and sisters provide help and support in caregiving (1.86)

b. Other members of the family help with caregiving demands (1.26)

c. Your parents help you with caregiving (1.56)

Response categories: (4) Very often; (3) Often; (2) Rarely; (1) Never.

E. Impact of caregiving demands on other activities (0.47).

From your personal experiences, please give your view on the following statements regarding your activities (work or in market).

a. Since the beginning of caregiving of this child, I have stopped other income generating activities (1.78).

b. I have changed my income generating activities since caring for this child (1.30).

c. My income generating activities have declined since caring for this child (2.55).

Response categories: (4) Completely agree; (3) Agree; (2) Somewhat agree; (1) Disagree.

F. Personal and social norms (0.78)

We have our personal and social norms that usually guide our thoughts and actions. In caring for a child living with HIV/AIDS, how do the following propositions apply to you?

a. Due to my age, I shouldn't be caring for a child at this point in time (1.50).

b. Due to my health, I shouldn't be caring for a child (1.41).

c. Other members of my family should be caring for this child (1.81).

d. Members of the other family should be caring for this child (2.18).

Response categories (4) Completely agree; (3) Agree; (2) Somewhat agree; (1) Disagree.

G. Impact of antiretroviral drugs (alpha = 0.90).

Antiretroviral drugs (ARVs) have improved the lives of people living with HIV/AIDS. Please answer the following propositions regarding your sentiments toward ARVs.

a. I have less worry now knowing that the child is on ARVs (3.15).

b. I have hope for the future of the child because he/she in on ARVs (3.04).

c. I think my hope for the child to grow can be realized because the child is on ARVs (3.17).

Response categories (4) Completely agree; (3) Agree; (2) Somewhat agree; (1) Disagree.

Table 2: Constructs and reliability (alpha) of each scale (Continued)

H. Supplemental efforts made for the child (alpha = 0.91)

Oftentimes caregivers make supplemental effort because of the illness of the person they care for. Please answer the following questions by circling the answer the best suits you.

a. I give more love to the child because of her/his condition (3.55).

b. I am more empathetic toward the child because of her/his condition (3.58).

c. I am more worried about the child because of her/his condition (3.75).

d. The child I am caring for is more spoiled because of her/his condition (3.39)

e. The child I am caring for is more special because of her/his condition (3.33).

Response categories (4) Completely agree; (3) Agree; (2) Somewhat agree; (1) Disagree.

I. Coping with stress (0.80)

Caregivers adopt some behaviors due to stress of caregiving. How often to you as a caregiver do this?

a. I stay alone by myself (2.00).

b. I put all in God's (3.66).

c. I avoid people (1.81).

d. I keep to myself (2.10).

e. I cry (2.41).

f. I take painkillers (1.49).

g. I read the Bible (Koran) (2.48).

h. I listen to religious songs (2.91).

i. I pray (3.48).

Response categories: (4) Very often; (3) Often; (2) Rarely; (1) Never.

J. **Positive comparison (alpha = 0.73)**

Below are some thoughts that caregivers of children with HIV/AIDS have. How often do you think these thoughts?

a. You try to remember qualities that you have appreciated from the child's parents (2.95).

b. You try to remember good times that you had with the child (2.94).

c. You try to remember good qualities that you had appreciated in the child (2.70).

d. You try to remember good times that you had with the child's parents (2.64).

Response categories: (4) Very often; (3) Often; (2) Rarely; (1) Never.

K. **Profound meanings of child's condition (alpha = 0.56)**

a. You try to find a reason for the condition of the child (1.59)

b. You say to yourself that the child has HIV/AIDS because of destiny (1.31)

c. You believe there is a reason behind the condition of the child (1.23)

Response categories: (4) Very often; (3) Often; (2) Rarely; (1) Never.

Concepts and their measures are explained above. Reliability (alpha) is calculated for each scale: N=201.

The disclosure scale has two subscales: (1)--family member and (2)--provider of help. The family member scale is a three-item scale that assesses whether or not caregivers had disclosed child's serostatus to her/his own family members, the family members on the other side, and the siblings of the child living with HIV or AIDS. The provider of help scale taps the fact that caregivers disclosed to only people they knew would provide them some type of help. In fact, they reported disclosing to people who could help them financially, emotionally, spiritually, or medically.

The expression of faith scale measures ways and frequency caregivers boosted themselves up when they were tired of the caregiving burden. It consists of five items: go to church, pray more, sing religious songs, listen to religious songs, ask to be prayed for.

The financial difficulties scale reports ways and frequency that caregivers financially fall short regarding caring for the child. Participants mostly reported not being able to: (1)--feed the child, (2)—provide clothing for the child, (3)—provide leisure for the child, (4)—provide sweet treats for the child.

The family support scale is a three-item scale that assesses the source and frequency of help that caregivers receive. It is noteworthy to report that since most caregivers did not disclose the child's serostatus to others, even family; they did not receive support from them. Also, those who disclosed the child's serostatus reported not receiving much support either.

The impact of caregiving demands on other activities scale stresses the impact of caregiving on caregivers' income generating activities. While some caregivers had stopped their income generating activities, most had seen these activities decline due to caregiving demands.

The personal and social norms scale has four items that depict caregivers' personal and social values about whether or not she/he should be caring for the child. Old age and health impairment were mentioned as being reasons why caring for the child was seen as inappropriate by caregivers.

The impact of antiretroviral drugs scale assesses caregivers' grateful sentiments for having the drugs for the children. For example, participants reported that they had less worry now that the child was on ARVs. They also stated that they had hope for the future of the child because of the ARVs.

Another scale consists of the supplemental efforts caregivers made for the child because of her/his condition. They, for instance, reported showing more love to the child living with HIV or AIDS, being more empathetic toward the child or spoiling the child, in a special way because of the child's condition.

Coping with stress is a nine-item scale. Caregivers reported staying alone, avoiding people, keeping to oneself, crying, taking painkillers, reading Holy Scriptures, listening to religious songs, praying, and/or putting everything in God's hands.

The positive comparison scale consists of four items that assess ways caregivers remembered qualities they appreciated in the child and the child's parents, as well as the good times they had with both the child and the child's parents. Finally, caregivers searched for reasons and profound meanings of the child's condition.

Conclusion

Measures of informal caregiving to children with HIV or AIDS in Togo were developed in this study. Eleven dimensions that describe caregivers' experiences were: 1) disclosure, 2) expression of faith, 3) financial difficulties, 4) family support, 5) impact of caregiving demands on other activities, 6) personal and social norms, 7) impact of antiretroviral drugs, 8) supplemental efforts made for the child, 9) coping with stress of caregiving, 10) positive comparison, and 11) profound meaning of child's serostatus. Although cross-sectional data were used in the study and some of the findings may change in longitudinal data, this study is a beginning effort to examine this important issue of informal caregiving to children with HIV/AIDS, especially in Africa.

The findings in this study are based on both qualitative and quantitative research as well as the author's research studies with informal caregivers of children with HIV/AIDS in Togo. As with any new instrument, it should be considered as a heuristic tool that will need additional research for further validation.

Acknowledgments

Fulbright Program with the African Regional Research Program supported this study. The author would like to thank all the people that made this study possible, especially caregivers who participated in the study.

References

Aranda, M.P. & Knight. B.G. (1997). The Influence of Ethnicity and Culture on the Caregiver Stress and Coping process: A Sociocultural View and Analysis. *Gerontologist*, 37:342-354.

Atkins, R. & Amenta, M.A. (1991). Family adaptation to AIDS: A comparative study. *Hospice Journal*, 7:71-83.

Bettoli-Vaughan, E., Brown, R.T., Brown, J.V., et al. (1998). Psychological Adjustment and Adaptation of Siblings and Mothers of Children with HIV/AIDS. *Families, Systems & Health*, 16:249-266.

Carlisle, C. (2000). The search for meaning in HIV and AIDS: The carers' experience. *Qualitative Health Research*, 10:750-765.

Derogatis, L.R., Lipman, R.S., Rickles, K., et al. (1974). The Hopkins symptom checklist (HSCL): A self-report symptom inventory, *Behavioral Science*, 19:1-15.

Family Health International (FHI). (2001). Care for orphans, children affected by HIV/AIDS and other vulnerable children: A strategic framework. Retrieved May 24, 2007, from http://www.fhi.org/en/HIVAIDS/pub/fact/carorphans.htm.

Folkman, S., Chesney, M.A., Cooke, M., et al. (1994). Caregiver burden in HIV-positive and HIV-negative partners of men with AIDS. *Journal of Consulting and Clinical Psychology,* 62:746-56.

Foster, G. (2000). The capacity of the extended family safety net for orphans in Africa. *Psychology, Health, and Medicine,* 5(1):55-62.

Foster, G. & Williamson, J. (2000). A review of current literature on the impact of HIV/AIDS on children in Sub-Saharan Africa. *AIDS*:14 (suppl 3):S275-S284.

Graffi, S. & Minnes, P. (1989). Stress and Coping in Caregivers of Persons with Traumatic Head Injuries. *Journal of Applied Social Sciences*, 13:293-311.

Horowitz, A.V. & Reinhard, S.C. (1995). Ethnic Differences in Caregiving Duties and Burdens Among Parents and Siblings of Persons with Severe Mental Illness. *Journal of Health and Social Behavior*, 36:138-150.

Land, H. & Hudson, S. (2002). HIV serostatus and factors related to physical and mental well-being in Latina family caregives. *Social Science & Medicine*, 54:147-159.

LeBlanc, A.J., London, A. S. & Aneshensel, C.S. (1997). The Physical Costs of AIDS Caregiving. *Social Science and Medicine*, 45(6):915-923.

Lesar, S., Gerber, M.M. & Semmel, M.I. (1995). HIV Infection in Children: Family Stress, Social Support, and Adaptation. *Exceptional Children*, 62:224-236.

Lesar, S. & Maldonato, Y.A. (1997). The Impact of Children with HIV Infection on the Family System. Families in Society: *The Journal of Contemporary Human Services*, 78:272-279.

McCubbin, H. I. & Thompson, A.I. (1987). *Family assessment inventories for research and practice.* (Eds.) Madison: University of Wisconsin-Madison.

Merson, M. & Rosenfield, A. (2000). *The AIDS Epidemic: Lesson Learned.* Lancet, 356:1204.

Moore, A.R. & Henry, D. (2005). Experiences of older informal caregivers to people with HIV/AIDS in Lomé, Togo. *Ageing International*, 30:147-166.

Moore A. R. & Williamson, D. A. 2003. Problems with HIV/AIDS prevention, care, and treatment in Togo, West Africa: Professional caregivers' perspectives. *AIDS Care*, 15:615-627.

Pearlin, L.I, Aneshensel, C.S. & LeBlanc, A.J. (1997). The Forms and Mechanisms of Stress Proliferation: The Case of AIDS Caregivers. *Journal of Health and Social Behavior*, 38 :223-236.

Pearlin, L.I, Mullan, J.T., Semple, S.J., et al. (1990). Caregiving and the Stress Process: An Overview of Concepts and Their Measures. *The Gerontologist* 30 (5):583-594.

Radloff, L.S. (1977). The CES-D scale: A self report depression scale for research in the general population. *Applied Psychological Measurement*, 1:385-401.

Seeley, J., Kajura, E., Bachengama, C., et al. (1993). The extended family and support for people with AIDS in a rural population in southwest Uganda: A safety net with holes? *AIDS Care*, 5, 121- 126.

Turner, H.A. & Pearlin, L.I. (1989). Issues of Age, Stress, & Caregiving. *Generations* 13:56-59.

UNAIDS/WHO. 2000. Epidemiological fact sheet. Geneva: UNAIDS, The Joint United Nations' Program on HIV/AIDS and the World Health Organization.

UNDP. 2006. Human development indicators: Country facts sheets. Togo 2006. Retrieved 3 March, 2007, from http://hdr.undp.org/hdr2006/statistics/countries/ country_facts_sheets_cty_fs_TGO.html.

UNESCO. 2007. HIV impact on education clearinghouse. HIV/AIDS in Togo. (Retrieved 3 March 2007, from http://hivaidsclearinghouse.unesco.org/ ev.php?ID=2840_201&ID2=DO_TOPIC.

UNICEF. 2002. Orphans and other children affected by HIV/AIDS. Retrieved May 24, 2007, from http://www.unicef.org/publications/pub_factsheet_orphan_en_pdf.

Wikipedia. 2007. Economy of Togo, available at: Retrieved March 3, 2007, from, http://en.wikipedia.org/wiki/Economy_of_Togo.

Index

B

C

D

G

H

I

J

K

L

M

N

O

P

Q

R

S

T

U

V

W

X

Y

Z